MW00562697

DMT
DIALOGUES

■ ■ ■ ■ ■

"*DMT Dialogues* represents an important step in the scholarly conversation about the DMT world and the entities which inhabit it. By presenting insightful contributions from experts in psychology, anthropology, religious studies, and neuroscience, as well as the interdisciplinary discussions that followed, the editors have provided the theoretical tools needed to start interpreting and understanding the DMT experience. As part of the Beckley/Imperial Research Programme we are currently investigating how DMT has its effect in the brain in a pioneering study using EEG and fMRI."

AMANDA FEILDING, FOUNDER OF THE BECKLEY FOUNDATION

"DMT is famous in the world of psychedelic research for inducing experiences that are short, a matter of minutes, but with effects that are profoundly dazzling and lead to lengthy essays that try to explicate the puzzle. It clearly affects the language centers of the brain! It has led to the recognition of DMT entities, which may or may not be a new class of weird beings, neither animal nor plant, molecular nor metaphysical. This book is a fascinating series of explorations of the paradigm-busting and mind-blowing experiences triggered by this substance. Just reading about them is mind-blowing!"

RALPH METZNER, PH.D.,
COAUTHOR OF *THE PSYCHEDELIC EXPERIENCE*
WITH TIMOTHY LEARY AND RICHARD ALPERT AND
AUTHOR OF *SEARCHING FOR THE PHILOSOPHERS' STONE*

"*DMT Dialogues* is a courageous attempt in the best tradition of the scientific process to wrestle with the meaning of anomalous DMT experiences, reported by a substantial number of people, involving the sense of being in touch with alien intelligences. Like all great mysteries, there is no single interpretation that everybody who participated in the *DMT Dialogues* arrived at by consensus. Reading *DMT Dialogues* will not bring you certainty but rather will bring you in direct contact with profound minds struggling to plumb the depths of consciousness."

RICK DOBLIN, PH.D., EXECUTIVE DIRECTOR OF THE
MULTIDISCIPLINARY ASSOCIATION FOR PSYCHEDELIC STUDIES (MAPS)

"Preserved in the pages of this book are some of the most extraordinary presentations I have ever had the pleasure to read. It was my privilege to attend the 2017 Tyringham Initiative DMT Symposium and to learn firsthand from the assembled scientists and scholars about their research into DMT. This substance opens doors into a hidden world, and to listen to—and read—these presentations is to discover that powerful advances are being made into understanding its meaning and potential."

WHITLEY STRIEBER, AUTHOR OF *COMMUNION* AND
THE SUPER NATURAL AND HOST OF *DREAMLAND* PODCAST

"*DMT Dialogues* showcases the incredible, groundbreaking work of the Tyringham Initiative, which convenes cutting-edge thinkers and scientists exploring the edge-realms of the psyche, with the intention of furthering humanity's understanding of what lies beyond the edge of the known."

DANIEL PINCHBECK, AUTHOR OF *BREAKING OPEN THE HEAD* AND
COFOUNDER OF REALITY SANDWICH AND EVOLVER.NET

"DMT has a rich cultural history, a radically vibrant contemporary social context, complex biological mechanisms, theological and philosophical implications, and far-reaching implications for the science of consciousness. In *DMT Dialogues*, David Luke and Rory Spowers have curated an accessible anthology that sparks off in many of these directions and then kindles them together into a Promethean fire for our times. Where do we go as a species with all this rising knowledge of the extraordinary farther reaches of the mind? Only time will tell, and I'm sure this book will help us find the way."

OLIVER ROBINSON, PH.D., AUTHOR OF *PATHS BETWEEN HEAD AND
HEART: EXPLORING THE HARMONIES OF SCIENCE AND SPIRITUALITY*

DMT
DIALOGUES

Encounters with
the Spirit Molecule

EDITED BY **David Luke** AND **Rory Spowers**

INTRODUCTION BY **Anton Bilton**

Park Street Press
Rochester, Vermont

Park Street Press
One Park Street
Rochester, Vermont 05767
www.ParkStPress.com

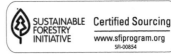

Text stock is SFI certified

Park Street Press is a division of Inner Traditions International

Library of Congress Cataloging-in-Publication Data
Names: Luke, David, editor. | Spowers, Rory, editor.
Title: DMT dialogues : encounters with the spirit molecule / edited by David
  Luke and Rory Spowers ; introduction by Anton Bilton.
Description: Rochester, Vermont : Park Street Press, [2018] | Includes
  bibliographical references.
Identifiers: LCCN 2017050203 (print) | LCCN 2017055063 (ebook) |
  ISBN 9781620557471 (paper) | ISBN 9781620557488 (ebook)
Subjects: LCSH: Hallucinogenic drugs. | Dimethyltryptamine. | BISAC: SOCIAL
  SCIENCE / Popular Culture. | MEDICAL / Psychiatry / Psychopharmacology.
Classification: LCC BF209.H34 D58 2018 (print) | LCC BF209.H34 (ebook) |
  DDC 154.4—dc23
LC record available at https://lccn.loc.gov/2017050203

Printed and bound in the United States by Lake Book Manufacturing, Inc.
The text stock is SFI certified. The Sustainable Forestry Initiative® program
promotes sustainable forest management.

10   9   8   7   6   5   4   3

Text design by Debbie Glogover and layout by Virginia Scott Bowman
This book was typeset in Garamond Premier Pro and Gill Sans with Delphin,
Noyh Geometric, and Hypatia Sans used as display typefaces.

To send correspondence to the authors of this book, mail a first-class letter to the
authors c/o Inner Traditions • Bear & Company, One Park Street, Rochester, VT
05767, and we will forward the communication, or contact the authors directly:
David Luke at **https://www.gre.ac.uk/eduhea/study/pswc/staff/dr-david-luke**,
Rory Spowers at **figtreediaries.com**, and Anton Bilton at
anton@tyringhaminitiative.com.

In Quest of Truth—seek truth, but remember that behind all the new knowledge the fundamental issues of life will remain veiled!

FROM THE TEMPLE OF MUSIC
AT TYRINGHAM HALL

CONTENTS

■ ■ ■ ■ ■

DAY ONE
The Origins, Evolution,
and Esoteric Culture of DMT

About the Entheogenic Plant Sentience Symposium

RORY SPOWERS

In September 2015, ten of the world's leading luminaries noted for exploring the mysterious compound dimethyltryptamine (DMT) gathered, along with a number of multidisciplinary discussants, in the United Kingdom at Tyringham Hall, the spectacular home of Anton Bilton, property developer and patron of consciousness research projects. Over three days, these open-minded explorers discussed the notion of entheogenic plant sentience and the role of DMT as a possible conduit between Spirit and Matter.

DMT Dialogues gives a potent distillation of the exchange of ideas among these leading thinkers from around the world—experts in archaeology, anthropology, religious studies, psychology, neuroscience, chemistry, and psychopharmacology. Presenters included Graham St. John, Dennis McKenna, Jeremy Narby, Peter Meyer, Erik Davis, Ede Frecska, Andrew Gallimore, Rupert Sheldrake, Graham Hancock, and Rick Strassman. Symposium attendees included Luis Eduardo Luna, Bernard Carr, Robin Carhart-Harris, David Luke, Jill Purce, Tony Wright, Will Rowlandson, Anton Bilton, Rory Spowers,

Vimal Darpan, Santha Faiia, Cosmo Feilding Mellen, Anna Hope, and Amanda Feilding.

This edited collection of presentations and discussions describes a wide spectrum of theories that have arisen within this field, ranging from the Simulation Hypothesis and the Multidimensional Universe to the possibility that DMT had ancient extraterrestrial origins. Others suggest that the chemical has played a prominent role in our cultural and religious evolution, from Paleolithic rock art, the Aboriginal Dreamtime, and the prophetic vision of the Old Testament through to the futuristic worlds of modern science-fiction films. What has emerged from this seminal meeting of minds is overwhelming evidence that DMT is somehow integral to the mediation between different states of consciousness, possibly even between life and death itself and, as a result, is worthy of rigorous investigation.

Through staging this event, the Tyringham Initiative was born, a world-class think tank or "Modern Mystery School" that believes the synthesis of Science and Spirit, and even direct experience of the divine, to be fundamental to reshaping our worldview. At a time when multiple scientific disciplines, from quantum physics to neuroscience, are converging on the core truth and mystic vision of the Perennial Philosophy—that Consciousness may indeed be primary and not secondary to Matter—the role played by a compound such as DMT seems ever more crucial to explore.

Could this next Copernican Shift in our understanding of Consciousness be the pivotal factor in helping humanity to reenvision its role in the universe and thereby take the necessary steps to make our political, social, technological, and economic systems synergistic with ecological parameters? And could our understanding of the role played by DMT prove to be the key to unlocking the great mystery of Consciousness itself? Perhaps the pages that follow will prove to be the start of us finding out.

Objectives
of the Symposium

DAVID LUKE*

DMT is a simple organic molecule present in an extremely wide range of animals and probably all plants, though curiously not fungus, which in true mycelial style has its own version: 4-HO-DMT. That DMT is also naturally occurring in humans is no doubt part of why it is so often experientially considered to be the strongest and strangest of all psychedelics, delivering half of all high-dose users to new yet curiously familiar alien worlds where sentient nonhuman beings await to greet them: "Welcome back, we missed you." Few experiencing these phenomena report anything less than a world seeming more real than this one.

Science explores, charts, navigates, discovers, and increasingly comprehends the physical world both macro and micro. It pushes the limits of outer space, yet is asleep at the wheel of our outward-thrusting vehicle, giving scant regard to mapping inner space, which is both within the universe and our personal container of it. And yet what could be a more important scientific research question in a materialistic world than locating, verifying, and communicating with beings apparently far

---

*Taken directly from the symposium program booklet for speakers and discussants.

more intelligent and knowledgeable than we are? Given that 100 million dollars has just been provided to boost the Search for Extraterrestrial Intelligence Research Project, also known as SETI, wouldn't we expect any project that already has half its researchers reporting positive communications equally if not more worthy of investigation? But where are all the research grants, the scientific papers, the scientists and experts? Ah, there you are! All ten of you, welcome back, we missed you!

The question of DMT beings, of plant sentience, of interspecies communication, of discarnate consciousness, of perhaps even dialoguing with the divine—these are surely some of the most important of all research questions. They cut to the heart of the nature of reality itself. The precise tool for this research has been available for more than fifty years, but the academy has left it in the pencil jar in the secretary's office, hiding in plain sight.

So what steps should be made on our road to discovery? What is the role of DMT in plant-human coevolution, and what is its origin? Can we verify this other world and these other beings? Is the DMT world just delusional? Is our imagination more tricksy and infinite than we give it credit for . . . or are these beings somehow real? If real, then what are their intentions, and what is our relationship to them? Is it time to establish an interdimensional embassy or to barricade our minds against "the other"? Or are we just finding a new way to dialogue with our (higher?) self? In any case, what can be learned from the beings and from DMT and our study of it, anthropologically, culturally, psychologically, linguistically, pharmacologically, medically, evolutionarily, heuristically, and epistemologically? Or does all this exploration just generate more questions than answers, a chimeric rabbit hole more labyrinthine than our crenulated brain will allow us to fathom and more obscure than dark matter? Maybe we will find out.

Acknowledgments

We would like to thank the following individuals for their help with the symposium: Max Baring for documenting it all on film; Lisa Laffague for helping smooth the way; Nikki Wyrd for the transcription of the talks and discussions; and all the staff of the Tyringham Initiative for looking after us.

■ ■ ■ ■ ■

The Origins, Evolution, and Esoteric Culture of DMT

The talks given on this day set the context for the symposium and examine where DMT came from, biochemically, as well as its role in the past, present, and future evolution of all species on our planet. Where it currently resides in contemporary literary and audiovisual culture is also described.

Curiosity and our quest for truth propelled us to consider what it is that the DMT entities are trying to tell us, as well as how this message is being incorporated into entertainment for the masses. Graham St. John, a cultural anthropologist, will trace how the presence of DMT has evolved culturally in film and music, becoming a household name. Dennis McKenna is known for his research in ethnopharmacology and ethnobotany, and his lecture and the ensuing discussion consider that there is no time like the present to explore the role of DMT and its entities in helping us understand the evolution of life and our relationship to our environment.

INTRODUCTION

Exploring Entheogenic Entity Encounters

ANTON BILTON

Entities, gods, aliens—they're certainly not new to us humans. For millennia man has been spoken to by beings, and our major religions, misguided or not, are based on these communions.

Today we are technologically advanced and can examine these visitations with a greater intensity than our ancestors. We can create experiments that provoke the communion, allowing us to see correlations in experiences, to gather evidence, to ask the entities for answers, to access their realms, and to act on their advice. To me this is the most important work we can do. Spending billions with NASA in a search for extraterrestrial life seems almost wasteful when we can spend a fraction of that and experience alternate sentient presences through consciousness-expanding practices as our ancestors did.

For what is life? We deem a biological and material body as imperative. Yet our conscious self may exist way beyond its occupation of our body. In one guise or another, most people believe this to be true.

One night, while traveling in the astral and provoked by a particularly sacred moment of a ceremony, words of humble gratitude spontaneously came out of my mouth: "Thank you for my existence."

It shocked me. Not my life, but my *existence;* and I saw the difference.

I've had many entity experiences. The first was at a very sad and difficult stage in my life when I was fifteen years old. It arrived, unprovoked, midmorning during a school break, and in a Saul-on-the-road-to-Damascus way, it was the most profound experience of my life. It triggered my interest in these messengers from the gods, and since then I've spent much of my time outside my business and family issues seeking ways to make contact with them.

Sometimes they're benign, sometimes apathetic, and sometimes malevolent. But perception is all, and frequently what one perceives to be demonic is also one's greatest teacher. To fear less and be fear-less seems to be the key to understanding.

An example of this was when a monstrous, horned, ten-foot-tall demon screamed down at me, his huge muscles rippling under his red and leathery skin: "You, you ignorant humans, you really think it goes you, then God. You're so bloody arrogant. Let me tell you, just as an ant is a god to a single-cell amoeba, and as a dog is a god to an ant, and as a man is a god to a dog, then it goes on in many, many more layers from man before one reaches the Godhead. The ant can destroy the amoeba; the dog can piss all over the ant's nest; the man can cut the dog's throat; and I can murder you. In that order, it's so simple. And yes, at the end there is the Cosmic Mind, pure consciousness, the "God" of everything, and we are all One, but between that and you there are layers and layers of what you call gods, and I'm just one of those. The ancient Egyptians, the Greeks, the Romans, all pagans, they had it right in their multigod beliefs but you, you've all gone way wrong with your single God theory. Now let me show you what I do as archdestroyer."

And he whisked me off my feet by the scruff of the neck and flew me away through a sky of planets to see the Shiva-esque chaos he had wreaked.

Wowzers! An introduction to the concept of *layering* and one that not only felt more real than real but also tweaked the intuitive truth button that lies embedded in one's gut. Layering: differing levels of intelligent beings way more evolved than us. Gods! Not God. Layers of gods. Some more powerful than others. All more powerful than us. Yet all, somehow, eventually or in the ever-present now, at one with the cosmic mind of all.

What is it with these demon teachers and their sermons that makes them feel so real?

Their perceived malevolence and our associated fear response seem purposefully designed to jolt one out of ego-based judgments and help one move into the fearless witness state.

What is it with all entity encounters that makes the meeting so profound?

Whether it's a prophetic vision, a near-death experience, an alien abduction, or an investigatory plant medicine/psychedelic trip, the interaction with an alternate sentient presence, an entity, always knocks one's socks off.

From tiny flying fairy-like nurses through translucent angels, geometric light beings, two-dimensional faceless plastic figures, snakes, vines, jaguars, alien Greys, talking play-school toys, machine elves, small-mouth huge-forehead humanoids, sexy succubi, coral-like plants, skeletal giants, burning blue light-saber flames, to the raging fleshy demon encountered above, these entities are purposeful, sentient, and intelligent. They know what they're doing.

In my view the aliens and entities we see today are the gods of our ancestors, and it's solely our greater understanding of technology that makes the difference, as the technology of today is the magic of past years. Just as the conquistadors were perceived as gods by the Indians, so all descriptions of gods and aliens lie solely in their perceived omniscience by their observer. If they're perceived as omniscient, then they're a god; if there's any notion of possible vulnerability, then they're an alien.

We could spend all day arguing about whether these entities exist. They have been as real to me as I am to myself while sitting here writing this introduction. Of course, perhaps that sense of my own reality might well be misplaced, but that's for later in this book, when we discuss ideas on the nature of subjective reality and our own place in it.

For now, let's go with the flow. Mankind has quested communion with our maker or our maker's minions since time immemorial. The religious scriptures and history books are packed with entity encounters. There's probably not a person on Earth who either hasn't had an encounter or doesn't know someone who has sensed an entity presence of one type or another. They're here! And it's nothing but our lack of proper fearless investigation into their existence and purpose that's holding us back from full-on communion. Nothing, that is, but their own complicity. Are they benevolent or malevolent, interested or disinterested, or simply sharing the stage?

Perhaps they're us from the future—highly evolved humans who have mastered time and space and are returning in time in an ethereal nonmaterial form to influence our development.

Perhaps they're gods and angels carrying out their creator's wishes.

Perhaps they're a super sophisticated alternate alien species scientifically observing us in the laboratory we call Earth just as we observe our subspecies in laboratories and zoos.

Perhaps they are farmers, tending their flock before a harvest!

Come what may, and given the vastness of the universe, it would seem churlish not to accept the possibility of other living entities whose forms may be as diverse from ours as we are to some of the living creatures on our own Earth. Just compare us to a giant jellyfish or the tiniest of bacteria.

We are forever trapped by our senses and the perceived confines of our temporal and spatial environment. What if parallel universes do exist, and access between those universes and our own has been mastered by beings unconstrained by material bodies?

If matter is just the pimple on the skin of existence, then imagine the freedom when unconstrained by its limitations. Imagine the freedom of operating in space—mind-space.

So where are we now? The ancients made every effort to commune with these entities; there was no greater work than dedicating one's life to sacred focus on communion with the gods and their emissaries.

Monotheism has outlawed these practices on penalty of death. Reductionist scientism has ridiculed them. (Yet weirdly, science accepts the notion of dreams without empirical evidence.) But too many people sense the presences. Whether it be by default or prayer, too many people know they're there in the shadows.

Our role is to bravely ignite this process, not with dogma or judgment but with open-minded investigation like the great explorers of old. After all, surely those adventurers who sailed on galleons over the supposedly flat horizon in search of a new world are no braver than our experimental-consciousness explorer taking a heroic dose of intravenous DMT or a heart-stopping injection of phenobarbital to achieve a sixty-second near-death experience prior to resuscitation!

We need to explore this arena. We need to test every conduit and pathway available to us. We need to listen to people who have had contact, and look for correlations in communions and visitations. We need to be open-minded and hopeful, not cynical. For what can be more important than seeking direction from communion with alternate sentient intelligences when our own intelligence is leading us to ecological destruction?

The ancients knew this and communed directly for advice. We must resurrect this process, objectively and with reverence, respect, and an open mind.

It's these thoughts that prompted me to work with David [Luke] and Rory [Spowers] in establishing the symposium on Entheogenic Plant Sentience at Tyringham, where great fearless scientific minds could share theories on what these entities could be and where they might be coming from.

I hope you find the explanations and ideas as startling, refreshing, and mind-blowing as I did.

It's time to accept that something's going on . . . and then humbly ask for help.

CHAPTER 1

The Pineal Enigma

Tɦe Dazzling Life anð Timeꝭ of
tɦe "Spirit Glanð"

GRAHAM ST. JOHN

The theme of my presentation is the pineal enigma, the dazzling life and times of the spirit gland. Essentially I'm interested here in drawing from aspects from my book *Mystery School in Hyperspace: A Cultural History of DMT,* which deals with the career of Rick Strassman's "spirit molecule" to tell how it has become a meme that has left the clinic and developed a life of its own. I'm sure this has been a surprise to many people, particularly Strassman.

The proposition that Strassman puts forward in his book *DMT: The Spirit Molecule* is based on his research at the University of New Mexico that took place over five years in the early nineties, where he had full approval to undertake the first human psychedelic study in the United States for a generation, in fact since Prohibition. He gave sixty volunteers a total of about four hundred separate injections of DMT, many of which were high doses. One of the key propositions that come out of Strassman's book is that the pineal gland is the producer of DMT, and this speculation that he addresses in the book has been received as factual, regardless of the reality that even today the pineal gland has not been established as producing DMT.

I'm interested in how this meme has impacted popular culture and esoteric circles. I think there's possibly no better place to start than Gaspar Noé's *Enter the Void*. It's a classic perverse epic and one of my favorite films. This is a scene from the opening segment of the film where the main protagonist, an American drug dealer named Oscar, smokes DMT [plays clip showing a person smoking DMT]. Shortly after this he's informed by a friend that smoking DMT enables a death trip, and not so long after that Oscar is shot dead in a dodgy Tokyo bar. The rest of the film involves Oscar undertaking a sort of Bardo-like journey between this life and the next, a perverse journey. One of the interesting things to me is that the director of the film, Gaspar Noé, was influenced by *DMT: The Spirit Molecule.*

One of the key and fascinating themes in this book is that Strassman undertakes a sort of loosely phenomenological approach to his subjects' experiences on DMT, and the book demonstrates a very faithful attention to the experiential reports of his volunteers. They have incredible visions and breakthrough events including blinding white light, timelessness, a feeling of unity, a sensation of dying and being reborn, and of course, contact with a range of entities.

Of significance for Strassman was that one of the positive effects reported by a significant number of volunteers resembled what is universally known as mystical experiences. These correlate with out-of-body experiences and near-death experiences and also have much in common with reported alien abduction phenomena. He condenses the experiences as a merger with, and I quote, "an indescribably loving and powerful white light that emanates from the divine, holy, and sacred." Not unlike those having a near-death experience, the receiver of DMT is, and I quote again, "embraced by something much greater than themselves or anything they previously could have imagined. The source of all existence. And those who attain this experience emerge with a greater appreciation for life, less fear of death, and a reorientation of their priorities to less material and more spiritual pursuits."

I just want to play a segment here from the film *DMT—The Spirit Molecule,* which was coproduced by Rick Strassman and directed by Mitch Schultz. This is Chris Meuli, one of the DMT volunteers:

I saw this city in the deep deep distance, it was dark green and there were many lights flickering and clouds flowing over it. And all this started after tremendous geometric patterns that are so incredibly rapid that you cannot describe it to anybody, they are so fast. After this slowed down I saw this city in the deep distance. So I was sort of watching that and then this ball of light got right past me, right in front of me, like "What was that?" It didn't scare me except it was so close.

After that I started looking around, and it's like you're in this place and you're going, "Why am I in this place?" And then I noticed there is this woman off to my right with a real long nose and green skin; she was turning this dial, and I realized she was turning the volume of lights up and down on the city in the distance. And as soon as I looked at her she noticed I was watching her and she said, "So what else do you want?" I said, "What else do you have?" She paused for little bit, got up, and came over to me and turned this sort of screwdriver and popped open the sides of my head, and I felt all this pressure release and I felt a lot better. And I thought, *that's odd,* because I felt fine before.

So that's one of many experiences that were recounted—some more than a decade later—by one of the volunteers. I believe there were about half of the volunteers who experienced entities of some description, a wide range of entities. There were mostly positive experiences, but there were also adverse experiences. I'm sure when we get into entities over the next few days that the range of experiential contact phenomena will be discussed.

The main idea in *The Spirit Molecule* concerns speculation on the functions of endogenous DMT. Strassman came to a proposition, or revelation, that since the effects of DMT appeared to mirror mystical and prophetic states throughout human history, such states could be mediated in the brain by way of the internal production and release of the so-called spirit molecule.

The metaphysics behind this proposition is that the pineal gland is the lightning rod of the soul, a gland mediating matter and spirit, brain and mind. That the pineal is integral to the transition between this life and the next by its excretion of large quantities of DMT at the moments of birth and death is a significant part of this idea, which hinges on a Tibetan Buddhist metaphysical framework.

When we die it is supposed that, and I'm quoting, "the life force leaves the body through the pineal gland, where a DMT release is speculated to be like the floodwaters carrying the soul to the liminal phase," or Bardo, between life and death as depicted in the *Tibetan Book of the Dead* and functioning as a kind of spirit antenna. For instance, pineal DMT release at forty-nine days after conception marks the entrance of the spirit into the fetus. The proposal that the soul is released to death from the region of the pineal is depicted in Alex Grey's wonderful painting *Dying,* which is featured on the cover of Strassman's book. We see here the painting depicts a dying human with vapor rising from the crown, all overseen by a spiraling pattern of multiple, disembodied, wide-open eyes [speaker shows a slide].

Now I'm going to make some very broad brushstrokes here, and I'm interested in placing Strassman's research at the beginning of the nineties and reviewing what was known at that time. He was intrigued by the status of DMT as an endogenous compound; that it was admitted passage across the blood-brain barrier suggested it had a natural role in the brain. From the mid-1950s a series of discoveries demonstrated that DMT and its close relatives are compounds that occur naturally in humans and other mammals. Since the 1950s, most research had focused on the possible role of DMT in psychopathologies, and among the chief interests was CIA mind-control research using psychedelics, cryptically named MKULTRA.

Since the mid-1960s however, a moratorium prohibited human research with DMT and other psychedelics. But at the same time we began to see research that speculated and established knowledge about the endogenous nature of DMT in humans. We had Julius Axelrod's paper in *Science* publishing findings that the enzyme indolethylamine N-methyltransferase (INMT) is capable of producing DMT in rabbit lung. By the 1980s, there was research looking into it as an endogenous hallucinogen. DMT is found everywhere in nature, and it's produced in the human body via a biosynthetic pathway originating with the essential amino acid tryptophan and its enzyme INMT.

With growing evidence of DMT's endogenous activity, it is conjectured that DMT is a neurotransmitter, and of special interest for Strassman was that precursor enzymes necessary for DMT synthesis had been found in the pineal gland. So he was basically working against the grain to speculate that "the body synthesized a compound with psychedelic properties that produced highly prized spiritual experiences, rather than highly maladaptive psychotic episodes."

I'm not going to go into great detail, because I'm not a scientist, but the pineal gland possesses vital functionality. It regulates the hormone melatonin, which it converts from serotonin, and a balanced melatonin cycle is essential for sleep, reproduction, motor activity, blood pressure, and immunity.

Although in early research Strassman investigated the role of the pineal gland's production of melatonin and its role in depression, he believed that the organ had a hidden psychedelic purpose. Interest in the psychedelic pineal gland was expressed in 1986 when he was invited to speak at Esalen. The hidden function of the pineal was later hypothesized in a 1991 issue of *Psychedelic Monographs and Essays* in which he identified the pineal as an enigmatic organ, shrouded in mystery. And I know that there are people here who could add something to this discussion in terms of Rick's arrival at this hypothesis, and I'm honored to be in the presence of those people.

Before I get into the cultural stuff, I'd like to speak just a bit on the pineal through history, the backstory. Rick Strassman's ideas about the psychedelic pineal did not emerge from nowhere. Descartes, the French philosopher, reckoned the pineal gland to be the seat of the soul. He meditated on this pinecone-shaped organ's role as a conduit for the soul. Esoteric philosophers have long made claims about the spiritual and paranormal propensities of the pineal, in particular its capacity, once activated, to enable psychic abilities: a sixth sense, powers of perception—especially those associated with vision—clairvoyance, seeing auras, being visited by entities, and being awakened to information from other dimensions.

The light-transducing ability of the pineal gland has led to its reception as the physical manifestation of the third eye, an idea traced to Hindu traditions, from which practices of meditation, yoga, and chakra balancing derive. The all-seeing eye can be traced to the ancient Egyptian symbol of the eye of Horus, which is recognized by occult historians as a precise graphic representation of a cross section of the thalamus and the pineal gland.

So I'm interested in at least two schools of thought about the pineal. One is loosely New Age and the other is gothic horror. For the New Age, loosely termed, the pineal is the key to higher consciousness and spiritual evolution. Helena Blavatsky, founder of the Theosophical Society, popularized the idea that a third eye belonging to our ancient ancestors had atrophied through the course of evolution into the pineal. For Blavatsky and contemporary esotericists, the reactivation of the pineal gland enabled lucid dreaming, out-of-body experiences, astral travel, and, ultimately, the evolution of consciousness.

This image [speaker indicates artwork on the slide] is one of the many synchronicities that I've experienced here, and I was glad to see that Luke Brown's depiction of Baphomet is in our program, at the back. His painting is a classic representation of this idea of the pineal being a key to higher consciousness, and we can see the key there in alignment with the sixth chakra and the pineal gland. We can see the depiction of the pinecone-shaped pineal at the top.

For some time we've seen an industry of underground research into the nature of the pineal gland, including practices to activate and decalcify your pineal and speculation concerning how yoga and meditation techniques can decalcify or detoxify it. A range of practices are said to stimulate the release of DMT from the pineal. Binaural beats, dark room retreats, light machines, and snuffs including "Pineal Flush," which is a rapé, which has a very penetrative piercing effect. Also among the products said to stimulate the psychedelic pineal is the Lucia N°03 Hypnagogic Light Machine, which is conjectured to produce DMT-like compounds in the brain.

That's broadly one tradition. The other tradition is that of gothic horror, where the key figure is H. P. Lovecraft, who envisions a cosmic horror show radically alternative to the Theosophical Society. In the fiction of Lovecraft, the pineal is an antenna that detects signals from the beyond. But it's not just an antenna—a stimulated pineal is proposed to let "them" in. Not the gateway to higher consciousness, but rather a stimulated pineal gland becomes a bridge to the dimensions favored by the Great Old Ones of the nihilistic Cthulhu mythos.

The key story here is Lovecraft's 1920 short story, "From Beyond." It's a story about a scientist who discovered the true function of the pineal gland, which is essentially malevolent. The pineal gland is stimulated by an electrical machine, making another dimension available to the senses. Not only are humans newly sensitive to another dimension in which entities dwell, but these entities, which appear like jellyfish monstrosities, also *see* humans who are now susceptible to their interventions.

This is a quote from one of the story's characters, Doctor Crawford Tillinghast, the scientist who's researching with this instrument: "We shall see that at which dogs howl in the dark, that at which cats prick up their ears after midnight. We shall see these things and other things which no breathing creature has yet seen. We shall overleap time, space, and dimensions and without bodily motion peer to the bottom of creation."

In 1986 there was a film adaptation of "From Beyond," directed by Stuart Gordon, which saw Lovecraft's concept truly animated. The film involves a resonating electromagnetic machine with a large tuning fork, which when activated awakens the sixth sense by way of the pineal and begins receiving abominations from the beyond.

Beyond that, the machine causes the abduction and disfigurement of scientists, who return with cannibalistic pineal-eating and sado-erotic appetites. Let me screen some footage from that film in which Tillinghast is now assistant to the mad Dr. Pretorius:

[Pretorius' private lab. The sonic resonator is switched on and Dr. Edward Pretorius has returned "from beyond" (after being decapitated), with a phallic-like protrusion on his forehead wiggling around and tentacles emanating from his grotesque fleshy body, one of which has Dr. Katherine McMichaels subdued in its grip. Pretorius addresses his former assistant Dr. Crawford Tillinghast.]

PRETORIUS: You are evolving into a being that has never existed before.

TILLINGHAST: *[Half naked and covered in blood, clutching his forehead, fighting the effects of the resonator.]* I'm Crawford Tillinghast!

PRETORIUS: Let it happen, Crawford. Let it out!

[Tillinghast is screaming in pain, clutching his forehead.]

McMICHAELS: Crawford!

[Tillinghast's forehead bulges, and finally a wiggling stalk of flesh shoots out. He is no longer screaming, and his new forehead protrusion is wiggling around and his first person visual perceptions are now very colorful and psychedelic.]

TILLINGHAST: Oh, it's so beautiful. So . . . beautiful!

PRETORIUS: Now you can truly see.

McMICHAELS: What have you done to him?

PRETORIUS: I only awakened his sleeping pineal gland. It did the rest itself.

So you get the idea.

[Audience laughter.]

For me there's an interesting resonance with the film *Fear and Loathing in Las Vegas,* which of course is based on the novel of that title by Hunter S. Thompson. The film offers something of an advancement on Lovecraft, while playing with a similar theme. Here it's not a resonating machine that opens the pineal, the gateway to the beyond, but rather a drug harvested from the pineal performs a similar function. Here's a scene from that film:

[Duke has just taken some "adrenochrome," and the effects are starting to kick in.]

DUKE: We should get some of that. Just eat a big handful and see what happens.

GONZO: Some of what?

DUKE: *[Spitting words.]* Extract of pineal!

GONZO: *[Staring at Duke with a strange smile.]* Sure. That's a good idea. One whiff of that shit would turn you into something out of a goddamn medical encyclopedia.

[Gonzo grows horns. His face becomes a Mexican demon mask.]

GONZO: Man, your head would swell up like a watermelon, you'd probably gain about a hundred pounds in two hours . . .

[A cloven hoof bursts through Gonzo's shoe.]

DUKE: Right!

GONZO: . . . grow claws . . . bleeding warts.

[Gonzo's chest expands, bony ribs bursting his shirt.]

DUKE: Yes!

GONZO: . . . then you'd notice about six huge hairy tits swelling up on your back . . .

[A tail lashes, hooves strike the floor.
Gonzo towers, a flame red demon.]

DUKE: Fantastic!

[Duke is now so wired that his hands are clawing uncontrollably at the bedspread, jerking it right out from under him. His heels are dug into the mattress with both knees locked, eyeballs swelling. Gonzo-demon looms against the ceiling.]

GONZO: . . . you'd go blind . . . your body would turn to wax . . . they'd have to put you in a wheelbarrow and . . .

[Gonzo's voice fades away. Duke's frenzied gaze reveals
Gonzo has reverted to normal human shape and size.]

GONZO: Man, I'll try just about anything; but I'd never touch a pineal gland.

DUKE: FINISH THE FUCKING STORY! What happened?! What about the glands?

This leads me into looking at the so-called DMT gland in popular culture and, particularly, in film. Pineal-produced DMT has appealed to scriptwriters of horror cinema who seek new devices to bridge the chasm between life and death. DMT provides new ways of exploring themes like possession and reanimation. A film like *Banshee Chapter* is an instant cult classic. It's a fabulous film, very complicated, deep, and convoluted. It's inspired by Lovecraft's "From Beyond," and the film adaptation weaves together Lovecraft's vision that an activated pineal is a bridge to the dark beyond with the knowledge that the pineal gland produces DMT and that state-funded mind control, specifically MKULTRA research by the CIA, has exploited this knowledge, with terrifying results.

Using a found footage approach, the fictional film narrates the tragic effects of what's called "DMT-19," which is extracted from human pineal glands in MKULTRA clinical research, with research subjects who are witness to malignant and threatening entities with long claws. Very deeply Lovecraftian-influenced themes.

This is an early scene from the film where the journalist, who disappears shortly after this scene, drops DMT-19 before he goes missing.

[James is in his living room talking to a camera to document his drug experience.]

JAMES: Hello. My name is James, and this little guy is 150 milligrams of specially enhanced dimethyltryptamine, DMT-19. It's supposedly impossible to find, but here I have it.

Now this film interests me for a variety of reasons, including the fact that clearly Strassman's meme—that DMT can be extracted from the human pineal gland—has strongly influenced the narrative. There has been a recent rush of horror films that have presented the role of DMT introduced into the body as enabling contact with the dead, which was exploited in the 2014 horror film *The Possession of Michael King*. After the tragic death of his wife, an aggrieved filmmaker and atheist sets about to make a film disproving the existence of life after death.

In one scene the main protagonist is in a graveyard at night, smoking DMT that was given to him by a necromancer.

[A laboratory. The mortician is dissecting a toad and extracting a gland while giving a commentary to Michael King, the atheist filmmaker.]

MORTICIAN: The Sonoran Desert toad contains dimethyltrypt-amine, or DMT, the most powerful psychedelic on the planet. The human body produces DMT. It's released when we die. It helps us pass to the other side. But taking it while we're still living simulates a near-death experience. I'm going to need to let it dry. Prepare it. It's gonna take some time. We need to wait until it's dark anyhow.

[Cuts to a cemetery at night where Michael and unseen cameraman meet the mortician who leads Michael in a DMT ritual.]

MICHAEL: *[to cameraman]* This novocaine is wearing off on my stomach, so this is starting to hurt like a bitch, man. Oh, there he is. *[to mortician]* Hey, sorry we're late. I got all turned around in here.

[The mortician has impaled a number of toads on spikes that are staked into the ground.]

MICHAEL: Jesus Christ. Did you kill these . . . did you kill these things?

MORTICIAN: The toads, their pain, agony, it creates this sort of energy that draws in the spirits. Assume the position. On your back.

MICHAEL: Right.

[Michael lies down between the impaled toads, and the mortician leans over him with a hookah pipe.]

MORTICIAN: The smell of burning DMT can be intensely nause-ating. Like burning plastic. *[Michael inhales the smoke.]* Now, as it takes effect, the world will shatter and your body will quickly fol-low. You may feel like you're starting to die, like you don't know how to breathe at all. But it's okay. You just need to let go and go with it. *[After inhaling, Michael's face contorts and his eyes roll back in his head. The mortician begins to perform a funeral ceremony, sprinkling soil on Michael as he looks up at him.]* To Almighty God we com-mend our brother Michael . . . and commit his body to the ground.

Ashes to ashes, dust to dust. *[The mortician now invokes someone else to take Michael's body.]* Roland Sykes. Roland Sykes, reclaim your physical body. Take this body . . . Shit!

[Suddenly a police siren is heard and torchlight appears.]

POLICE: You, hey!

[Clip ends. Audience laughter.]

I'm not sure whether this film is supposed to be horror or comedy, but for me it was neither scary nor funny. It's a bad film for a whole bunch of reasons, including the fact that clearly there's misinformation concerning the Sonoran Desert toad being the source of DMT rather than 5-MEO-DMT, and I'm not sure what's going on with those toads either.

Another more recent film is *The Lazarus Effect,* where pineal DMT is the base compound for a serum called Lazarus that, you guessed it, brings back the dead. Here's a scene involving the two scientists in the film, discussing their differing views on the role of the pineal:

[Medical researchers Frank and Zoe are explaining
"the science" to the videographer Eva.]

FRANK: You know what the pineal gland is?

EVA: No.

FRANK: It produces DMT, which is the base compound for our serum. Basically, nobody knows why, but the moment you die, right then, your brain just floods your system with this massive blast of DMT, which is the most potent psychedelic on the planet. And when you think you're seeing the light at the end of the tunnel or the blessed Virgin Mary *[makes a sign of the cross]*, um . . . Did I do that the wrong way?

ZOE: Mm-mm.

FRANK: Anyway, it's just a big trip that you're having; really, it's all it is.

ZOE: I disagree. I do.

FRANK: Oh, you disagree, really? We've had this discussion before.

ZOE: Yeah, I just think you can't discount every near-death experience based on one theory.

FRANK: Of course. But if you're going to make a bet, why not bet on a scientific theory as opposed to, you know, St. Peter and the pearly white gates?

ZOE: Why?

FRANK: Because one is empirical and one is, you know, it's a cute story, but it's . . .

ZOE: No, it's not. I mean, whatever you wanna' call it, the soul, consciousness, it's just neural impulses firing in your brain, right? That makes it energy. Energy can't be created or destroyed, it can just be transformed from one thing to another. So that's not superstition, that's science.

EVA: So what's your theory?

ZOE: I think, maybe when we die, the DMT is there to help our souls move on, to get them wherever they're supposed to be. You know, open the door for them.

FRANK: So the DMT is like a doorman who is like, "Here. Here's life, here's death. I'm gonna open this up and usher you through."

ZOE: Maybe.

FRANK: And you give him a tip.

ZOE: I just think it's arrogant to reduce everything that happens at the moment of death to one chemical equation. The fact is, we just don't know.

FRANK: Yet.

While these scientists disagree about what transpires when pineal DMT floods the brain, there's no argument that something happens when you die, and DMT is there to lubricate the event. After the research team finds success with the DMT serum by reviving a dead dog, Zoe, one of the scientists who just happens to die in an electrical accident in the lab, is then reanimated with dark paranormal abilities that she uses to slay the other members of the research team. Here, pineal DMT provides a fresh means of replaying the tragic consequences of conquering mortality that have been a staple of sci-fi horror since Frankenstein.

And now for something completely different. I have to actually thank David Luke for providing me with a tip on this particular piece from the children's animated television series *Adventure Time*. It just demonstrates that this meme shows up in the unlikeliest of places, even reaching into children's animated television with decidedly adult themes. Here's Finn, from that series.

[Finn is onstage at a science conference organized for Princess Bubblegum and her guests.]

FINN: Ladies and gentlemen, and Princess, I'm here to talk about multidimensional bubbles. I'm not just going to talk about blowing bubbles, I'm going to blow . . . your . . . minds! This *[produces bubble maker]* is a bubble maker of my own design. This can blow bubbles in different dimensions. *[Finn starts the maker creating bubbles of different dimensions.]* This two-dimensional bubble has a one-dimensional shadow. This three-dimensional bubble has a two-dimensional shadow. *[On the final setting, a gyrating tesser-*

act bubble emerges.] This fourth-dimensional bubble casts a three-dimensional shadow. It is beyond comprehension! It is beyond space, beyond time!

PRINCESS BUBBLEGUM: Finn, that would mean you've created . . .

FINN: Yes, a black hooooole!!

[A black hole appears behind the stage and starts sucking everything in. Jake quickly extends his bendy arms and secures himself to the posts catching everyone and preventing them from getting sucked in along with the furniture.]

PRINCESS: Finn! Do something!

FINN: Don't worry, I have everything under control.

PRINCESS BUBBLEGUM: Under control? My guests are terrified.

FINN: Yes, and their brains are releasing adrenaline, dopamine, even dimethyltryptamine from their pineal gland! This has serious educational value. Thanataphobia and this NDE is giving us euphoric altered awareness. Don't you see, Princess, we were all BORN TO DIE!!

PRINCESS BUBBLEGUM: Are you trying to kill us all?

FINN: No of course not, I'm trying to give you the greatest conference EVER!

It was David who recited that to me at Breaking Convention in 2013. I don't know how he did that—he must have been listening to it on play loop.

Now to the spirit molecule in music. I was taking a look at Discogs recently, where I observed over thirty tracks entitled "Spirit Molecule." While there are representations from across genres, most are psychedelic trance. There are tracks, for example, offering the voice of Joe Rogan, who's probably the second most sampled individual in the spectrum of psychedelic electronica, with Terence McKenna, of course, being the most sampled person by far, and continues to be so in contemporary productions such as the track "Liquefied" from Hujaboy, and Quantize's remix of LOUD's track, "Dymethyltryptamine" (*sic*).

These are examples of what I've been calling "nanomedia," which are audio fragments from popular culture, film, altered statesmen like Rogan here, and of course Terence, and many others, that are programmed into tracks and played by DJs for the interactive theater of the dance floor. These samples are dropped into breaks in the music and become fascinating ways in which popular interests are absorbed and played with. One such track is called "Spirit Molecule" by Wizack Twizack, in which there is a sample referring to a strange chemical with the capacity to replicate an experience identical to events to come after life.

But psychedelic trance music is not the only music that has received and carried this meme. LA heavy metal outfit DMT is one such band. Bass player and founding member Alistar Valadez acknowledges the influence of *DMT: The Spirit Molecule* in public statements, where he has commented that DMT is a gateway to higher dimensions or astral realms.

Even country artists are getting in on the act. Released in 2014, Kentucky singer Sturgill Simpson's "Turtles All the Way Down" conveys an indebtedness to DMT and Rick Strassman in a struggle with faith reminiscent of Johnny Cash.

> *There's a gateway in our mind that leads somewhere*
>   *out there beyond this plane*
> *Where reptile aliens made of light cut you open and*
>   *pull out all your pain*
> *Tell me how you make illegal something that we all*
>   *make in our brain*

*Some say you might go crazy but then again it might
make you go sane*

*Every time I take a look inside that old and fabled
book
I'm blinded and reminded of the pain caused by some
old man in the sky
Marijuana, LSD, Psilocybin, and DMT
They all changed the way I see
But love's the only thing that ever saved my life*

So you saw it here first: psychedelic country! I'm not sure where to go from there!

In 2013, Rick Strassman coauthored a paper reporting that DMT has been found in the pineal microdialysate of live rats. It's an important step in the trajectory of this research, but no research yet proves that the pineal produces DMT. Is the pineal gland a threshold between the material and spiritual worlds, complete with a substance that fuels the transit?

Spirit gland? Sorcerous portal? The key to higher consciousness? A menacing doorway to the beyond? Or something decidedly more mundane? The pineal gland is a most enigmatic organ, and I look forward to continuing to research this phenomenon. Thank you.

DISCUSSION OF
The Pineal Enigma: The Dazzling Life and Times of the "Spirit Gland"

ANDREW GALLIMORE: What I found particularly interesting when you were talking about Lovecraft is that story was written in what, 1920?

GRAHAM ST. JOHN: 1920, yes.

GALLIMORE: So this is way before DMT was even known to be psychedelic, certainly way before there was any information that people might be secreting it, so how did Lovecraft get the connection that the activation of the pineal gives rise to bizarre entities? That seemed like a very strange coincidence that he would come to that conclusion, unless he had some sort of insider knowledge from these Mystery schools or something like that. Explain that.

ST. JOHN: Well I'm not sure that I can explain it; it is a fascinating development, and it's something that, as I said, I haven't written about—it's fresh data for me. It's interesting to compare this gothic horror trajectory with the trajectory of the Theosophical Society. I think that's interesting, but there's also deeper roots to this. I guess you could look at the way ancient Egyptians approached the pineal gland. I don't think there's a great deal of research on that, but there's a lot of speculation concerning what the Egyptians were doing with the pineal gland.

GALLIMORE: What did they know? You know, that's the interesting question. There's no reason that you would suddenly jump from "the pineal is the third eye" to, say, "when you activate it you see strange disembodied intelligences that attack you," you know? I mean to me that's a completely incomprehensible leap unless Lovecraft had some inside knowledge.

GRAHAM HANCOCK: Can I just add to that? Because there was an eye-opening moment for me. Now, Dennis [McKenna], I don't know how much you stand by this, but the identification of *Acacia nilotica* as the ancient Egyptian Tree of Life is intriguing, it's really intriguing, because that's a DMT-bearing tree.

DENNIS MCKENNA: Yes it's a DMT-bearing tree, and interestingly enough, the Masai use it as a potherb—they cook with it. But there's no indication they're even aware of the psychedelic properties, because there's no monoamine oxidase (MAO) that's activated; so this is interesting.

HANCOCK: Could it be that the DMT from the Tree of Life was inhaled by the ancient Egyptians?

McKENNA: Yes, that seems most likely.

HANCOCK: You were making this point about what the Egyptians knew of the pineal, and for me when Dennis made this species identification of the tree—that's a revelation. When you see the role of the Tree of Life, its connection to life beyond death, the idea of immortality, pharaoh's name being written on the Tree of Life, and finally we realize this is a DMT-bearing tree—extraordinary!

GALLIMORE: Yes, but there's still no clear link; they seem like parallel issues. I mean how would they link the pineal to the production of DMT? Or these entities? That to me . . . it's one thing to consume a plant that contains DMT, but how do you then link that to the pineal?

ST. JOHN: Of course Lovecraft wasn't talking about DMT.

GALLIMORE: He wasn't, no.

ST. JOHN: So what's fascinating is how this meme, this theory of the spirit molecule and the idea that the pineal produces DMT's psychedelic properties, has been adopted to enhance these stories in contemporary horror.

ERIK DAVIS: I guess that the somewhat less razzle-dazzle way of telling the story is just that from Descartes on, there's been an association of the pineal as a threshold between matter and spirit. This association gets taken up by Theosophy in the late nineteenth century and therefore plugged in to ideas of the astral realms and other dimensions and higher beings. Lovecraft is just inverting the signs—is taking the positive thing and switching it. So if you're Lovecraft and you want to look at the human body and you want to figure out "what's going to bring in my alternate baddies?" then that's the one you would go to. I think that part of what Graham's story is really more about is what Strassman invoked when he made that speculation. So when he makes the speculation, he's thinking about it on one level biologically, and how we could account for these processes, but by saying the pineal he's also invoking this whole cultural tradition that then goes on and kind of runs with it, almost beyond his control.

DAVID LUKE: There's some interesting coincidences paralleling that. Lovecraft's source material was his dreams, right? He was having these kinds of experiences that he then converted into these horror stories; so he did have some kind of direct access perhaps, some insights.

DAVIS: Yes. One other point on that is that it was also interesting the way that you [Andrew] perhaps unconsciously replicated one of the tricks that's already embedded in the Lovecraft mythos, which is to say, "Well, he clearly must have been connected with some kind of Mystery school," which for him is particularly ironic because he was a staunch sceptical materialist in all of his communications, so it's a kind of funny thing to accuse him of. And yet that's also something that's very much part of the Lovecraftian current, which is to suspect that there's some other source or some kind of questionable influence.

McKENNA: Perhaps that's why his dream life was so active, because he was a staunch materialist and yet he had this intuition that just beyond the threshold were these experiences.

DAVIS: Absolutely.

McKENNA: I hope it wasn't like it was depicted in the movie for him, or I feel sorry for the man.

DAVIS: They were mostly nightmares.

LUKE: I think Rupert and Ede have something to ask.

RUPERT SHELDRAKE: Well, yes, in 1984 I was in Esalen with Rick Strassman and Terence McKenna etcetera, and both Rick and I took

DMT for the first time, with Terence, and it then led to a series of conversations. I started my career as a tryptophan biochemist; my Ph.D. thesis was on the breakdown of the amino acid tryptophan, and I discovered that in plants when tryptophan breaks down as part of a dying process, it releases indole acetic acid, known as auxin, which is the main plant hormone. Auxin is a breakdown product of tryptophan. Another breakdown product is tryptamine and its derivatives, like DMT. So we were discussing the breakdown of tryptophan in dying cells, and the idea was that in the pineal there'd be these tryptophan precursors, and the pineal, at the moment of death, could flood the brain with DMT. This is a speculation Rick and I came up with in a conversation. I was amazed to see how far it's gone!

[Audience laughter.]

MCKENNA: You have to watch those morphogenetic fields.

[Laughter.]

SHELDRAKE: Well, I remember having these discussions with Rick at the time on how we could actually test this, and my idea was going to slaughterhouses, where they're killing animals anyway, and simply rapidly extracting the pineal gland from the brains of cows, pigs, sheep, etcetera, and freezing it—putting it in liquid nitrogen—and doing a DMT analysis. Well, we had this idea, neither of us got 'round to going to slaughterhouses and collecting pineal glands, but it's still a good idea.

[Audience laughter.]

It wouldn't be difficult to do. The brain would undergo any change that's happening anyway, so the animal rights people won't be especially upset because they're slaughtering the animals anyway, and it did seem to me a simple way to test this hypothesis. But it seems that most people don't actually need much of a test, it just seems to have taken on a life of its own.

JILL PURCE: I'd just like to say, Rupert's being very modest. I was there at the time, and actually it was Rupert who suggested it.

VIMAL DARPAN: Why hasn't this been tested?

SHELDRAKE: Well, because I suppose analyzing the DMT would require thousands of pounds, thousands of permits. How many people would risk their career in a lab, etcetera? You know it's still incredibly easy to do, collecting pineal glands from slaughterhouses, and nowadays there are all sorts of labs where you can send samples along and have them analyzed by gas chromatography or mass spectroscopy. And it may not just be the pineal. When cells die, they give off compounds they don't produce when they're alive; that's how plant hormones are produced, they're produced in dying cells. As the wood cells in the stem form, they break down—they commit suicide—and they give off plant hormones that cause more growth. So this may well happen in dying brains. Anyway, that was what I described. I'm amazed at how much progress there's been in the realm of the arts and how little progress there has been in the realm of science since then.

[Laughter.]

LUKE: I know Rick's not here personally, but I think there was some research actually done—he managed to extract pineal glands from cadavers. Is he back?* Is that right, Rick? But I don't think they found anything, particularly because the glands weren't fresh frozen and there may have been time for them to degrade. Rick, can you fill us in on that?

RICK STRASSMAN: So when I was doing my DMT study, I began to work out an underground project with the board of medical examiners for the county and collected a number of cadavers' pineal glands from recently deceased humans, and I sent those to be analyzed for DMT,

---

*Rick Strassman joined each presentation and discussion via Skype.

but none was found. So chances are that because the glands weren't fresh frozen the DMT degraded.

I don't know if you have mentioned while I was offline that it is now known that DMT occurs in the living pineal gland. There's a group in Ann Arbor, Michigan, led by Steve Barker, that has a very sophisticated means of looking at the pineal gland, and they determined that in the living rodent pineal gland there is DMT. And so that's consistent with the pineal production of DMT, even though locating the compound in that organ doesn't necessarily mean it's produced there.

The enzyme that metabolizes the synthesis of DMT, the N-methyltransferase, is found in high levels in the pineal in the rhesus monkey, and also the gene that codes for that enzyme is expressed to a large degree in rhesus monkey pineal. So that is quite strong circumstantial evidence: the enzyme is present, the genetic apparatus that synthesizes the gene is present, and the DMT itself is present even though it's in a different species—the monkey for the genetic data and the rodent for the DMT data. I suppose if you radio labeled the precursor you would probably have some ideas about that, if you found that DMT actually is being synthesized in the pineal.

The same group in Ann Arbor, Michigan, is looking at the dying brain to determine if concentrations of DMT increase in our brain, and that paper recently came out in the *Proceedings of the National Academy of Sciences,* and the scientists couldn't find any DMT in the dying brain. There are high concentrations of serotonin. But strictly speaking, serotonin isn't a precursor of DMT.

LUKE: Thanks for that, Rick. Good to see the research did actually happen, although probably not in the best circumstances. There's a need to get fresh cadavers. Ede, you had a point you wanted to make.

EDE FRECSKA: Yes. Three things quickly. So Steve Barker detected DMT in the pineal gland; the question is, how to stimulate the pineal gland, how to increase the level of DMT. There is a possible way—sonic stimulation. This is what monks do when they focus the "om" on the third eye. It's a very fragile but possible way. And easily detected—take a pig and put sonic waves on its head, and you can possibly find the increase if it is true. The study of sonic stimulation is very simple and easy and doesn't need too much money. My second point is about dreams and the pineal. You know that Descartes based his philosophy on three dreams; that was the source of his philosophy, he admitted it. And third, tomorrow I will discuss how the lung can be a possible source that floods the brain with DMT.

PURCE: Can I just add to that? With the overtone chanting, which is what the monks do, the method of doing it is to press the tongue up toward the roof of the mouth, pressing the air right up into the direction of the pineal gland.

FRECSKA: So we can do something similar by using sonic waves in experimental animals. Pigs because they are big enough.

PURCE: But maybe they can't overtone chant?

[Laughter.]

FRECSKA: I will do it with a sonic generator.

LUKE: Of course in that clip in the Lovecraft film where the man's pineal gland pops out of his head, they were using sonic resonators to activate the pineal gland—just to apply some warning.

MCKENNA: I just wanted to ask Ede a question. You're familiar with Jace Callaway's theory that DMT modulates dreams, and there's this whole cycle with melatonin and the day/night cycle. Cerebrospinal concentrations of DMT gradually increase over the night as you get into deep dream states. Is there any possible experimental approach to test the DMT levels and confirm it? Not that anyone will fund this kind of thing, but is it practical to think that you could? It's a very interesting hypothesis; could you put evidence under that hypothesis?

FRECSKA: There is one method, you know: PET scan?* You could give the precursor, and you make that precursor act in a certain part of the brain by PET scan. That's the only way.

LUKE: I did a very indirect experiment on this hypothesis actually, looking at dream extrasensory perception (ESP) and melatonin cycles, with peak melatonin occurring at three a.m. We actually woke people up at three o'clock in the morning and got them to do dream ESP tasks and compared their performance with their performance at eight a.m., assuming that DMT is perhaps a good modulator or trigger to dream ESP. There were significant positive results in the first experiment, but it didn't replicate. Obviously this is a very indirect proxy measure of possible nocturnal DMT production and dream modulation and a vague stab at Callaway's DMT dream hypothesis. It's a long way from a direct measure.

STRASSMAN: Concentrations of DMT are still really hard to measure in the endogenous state, and it may turn out that we need to look at nitrogen oxide concentrations, which when we pretreat with a mono-amine oxidase (MAO) inhibitor are significantly higher than the parent compound. A few months ago a grad student at UC Berkeley ran a little study by giving a monoamine oxidase inhibitor to a group of normal volunteers to determine if you could find measurable levels of either the parent compound or the oxide. And she unfortunately didn't measure the degree of monoamine inhibition, but nevertheless we weren't able to determine, or weren't able to detect, levels of either the anoxide or the parent compound. Like after you drink ayahuasca, the concentrations of the anoxide are quite a bit higher than the concentrations of DMT. So it could be that if you're looking at circadian rhythms of DMT synthesis in the dream cycle, then you may need to pretreat with an effective dose of the mono amine oxidase inhibitor.

Also an interesting point that hasn't really been looked at is that

---

*Positron emission tomography scan

there is a small number of people whose pineal glands have been destroyed by a stroke or a tumor, and the only thing that was abnormal about those people was they may not have been able to accommodate as readily to jet lag as people with pineal glands. But whether they dream normally or have the same frequency of spiritual experiences has not been looked at, as far as I know. If you have a large enough population there would be a handful of people without pineal glands, so that would be interesting. But obviously if the primary source of DMT is the lungs, then the pineal may just kick in at special times.

TONY WRIGHT: Regarding the DMT-dream theory, I had a lot of experience in the mid-nineties with extreme sleep deprivation. I was doing a lot of experiments of three to five and even seven days, and I had repeated windows of DMT-like experiences, including extreme and orgasmic euphoria and all kind of associated experiences. I've no idea what my biochemistry was like or anything like that, but it wouldn't be difficult to test. It's an ancient approach to altered states, so it may be that you force yourself beyond the normal circadian rhythms and other stuff starts to happen. Obviously I did it with research initially, but eventually it became quite addictive. Many people thought I was torturing myself, but actually I was having a great time once I got through the initial tiredness.

LUKE: Good pioneering work. There is some speculation as well, of course, about the Kogi Indians, in their use of light deprivation. They divine whether each new child born is going to become a shaman in the community, and those selected are put in a cave, where they grow up for the first nine years of their life and they have a very limited exposure to external light sources. There is some speculation that that may also have some effect on pineal gland development and melatonin and possibly DMT production. Yes, Rick.

STRASSMAN: On the question of whether the pineal is involved in spiritual-like experience in continuous darkness, there is evidence that the pineal atrophies in continual darkness. If you wanted to determine if DMT levels increase in accordance with dark phenomena, I would encourage you to give an effective dose of MAO inhibitor and collect urine. I don't know much about how we're living [lifestyle] can turn the transcription of genes into enzymes, but if there were a way to assess the activation of the gene responsible for indolethylamine N-methyltransferase (INMT) synthesis, then you could introduce continuous darkness and perhaps have a sensible way to determine activation of that system.

McKenna: Your mention of pineal tumors, Rick, is very interesting because it reminds me of a story, an anecdote. I don't know if there's evidence for it, but Alex Grey's assistant was telling me about a person who apparently had a pineal tumor where the cells were proliferating. You mentioned that a tumor would probably destroy pineal function, but apparently in this case, if there's any truth to this story, it actually hyperactivated pineal function, and this person was in a visionary state all the time. He was dealing with that by becoming a very highly talented visionary artist. Have you heard anything about this? What do you think? Is that just a wild tale, or is there any basis to it?

Strassman: Well, it's a truly wild tale, but it's true. The guy's name is Shawn Thornton, and he started sending me paintings of his maybe ten years ago. I told Alex about this guy and sent Alex some of his paintings, and they're quite DMT-like. They're not as visionary as Alex's paintings, with their morphing buzzing visual geometric pattern; Shawn's are more intricate. He had all of these visions while he was suffering from the tumor. After the tumor was removed he stopped having those visions but was able to remember what his experiences were like while the tumor was there, and he continued painting. He's still painting, and he began to show his work in galleries.

McKenna: So it's a real tale. I didn't just dream this up somewhere. It's not a false memory! That's very interesting.

PURCE: I'd like to say Alex Grey and I had the same Tibetan teacher. I've been studying with him for over forty years, and in Tibetan Buddhism the ultimate path is what's called the rainbow body, which is the transformation of flesh into light at the moment of death—Jalü. And the two practices that lead up to this, thödgal and the dark retreat, are both practices related to light. One is a form of looking at light, looking at the sun, which is done for long periods. And the other is dark retreat, which elicits what they call the inner light, so that there's a combination of the inner and the outer light. So extended periods of complete dark retreat are an essential part of this practice for the transition into the body of light.

LUKE: A bit like the Kogi then in many respects.

PURCE: But highly sophisticated, highly organized, and well known; yes.

MCKENNA: It seems like we couldn't really put any of this to the test until we have a reliable way to bioassay and analyze for DMT in the living organism. I guess you would sample cerebrospinal fluid; would that be the most obvious place? Continuously through a catheter or something like that, you would have to be able to catch this in real time and then . . .

GALLIMORE: They have far more functional magnetic resonance imaging (fMRI) technologies now. It's possible to have highly detailed high-resolution pineal images that light up in the presence of DMT.

MCKENNA: What's the limit of detection?

GALLIMORE: Well, it's improving. But fMRI, you know. Excellent detectability anyway.

MCKENNA: So in a few years we'll be able to answer this question.

GALLIMORE: Yes, yes. It's an emerging field now, pharma-fMRI.

LUKE: Well, one of the questions that comes up, though, is, What's a suitable quantity to have an endogenous DMT experience from pineal DMT if we detect it? Given that the pineal gland weighs 144 milligrams itself, perhaps a lot of that would have to be DMT if we're talking about the same kind of dosages as for smoking DMT or injection. So one would have to assume the endogenous doses would be somewhat smaller, or is a third of the pineal gland made up of DMT?

LUNA: Jace Callaway objected to the possibility of the pineal gland releasing enough DMT to produce any experiences. The tiny amounts will not be enough.

LUKE: But we don't know what the dosage is endogenously. One would assume that it'd be far less than smoking it, but it's hard to say, isn't it?

McKENNA: The real question is, What is the concentration at the synapse? Probably most of the DMT that you take exogenously is destroyed before it ever gets to the synapses, so maybe 10 percent of your 50 milligram dose, if that much; I mean Ede, what is your thought on that?

FRECSKA: Really, it depends what is channeling the DMT, so definitely if it would be humoral, then there is some serious doubt whether the concentration is enough. But if there are certain pathways that would deliver the DMT to a certain part of the brain involved in dreaming, that can be a different picture.

LUKE: I think we're going to draw to a close now for this session, so thank you, everybody, for participating. Thank you very much, Graham.

CHAPTER 2

Is DMT a Chemical Messenger from an Extraterrestrial Civilization?

Dennis McKenna

I perhaps made a mistake when I suggested this topic, "DMT: A Chemical Messenger from an Extraterrestrial Civilization." I was at a place where the abstract was due, so I more or less put the title up and then I wrote an abstract around that, and then I actually started to put together the talk. So what you're going to find is that the abstract and the talk don't bear that much relation to each other. But hopefully it will be interesting. So here it goes.

What do we know about DMT? Well, there are a few things that we have pretty well nailed down. We are very familiar with what its chemical characteristics are—it's *N,N*-dimethyltryptamine, it has a much longer chemical name, it's one of the simplest indole alkaloids and perhaps one of the simplest tryptophan derivatives that's found in nature. We know what its chemical properties are, and that's maybe the takeaway from this slide—that it's extremely simple. It was actually first synthesized by a Canadian chemist, Richard H. Manske, in 1931, who was working on of all things the constituents of strawberry roots. He needed some standards for chromatography, so he synthesized dimethyltryptamine. It was not known at the time that it was a natural compound, so he assumed it was synthetic. He synthesized it, did his chromatography, put it on the shelf, and it was forgotten for ten years. He had no idea that it was psychoactive. But he deserves the credit for being the first person that actually synthesized it. Manske went on to become famous for his work in alkaloids and edited a multivolume series called *The Alkaloids*.

The pharmacology of DMT is known to you from theory and also from objective sources. We know that it's generally short acting when it's taken parenterally; when it's not taken through the stomach, it lasts a very short time. It's a true psychedelic under the framework that I like to define, which is that it's an endogenous 5-HT_{2A} agonist as well as a 5-HT_{1A} agonist, and it interacts with other receptors as well to produce a psychological response. But 2A agonism is the accepted characteristic of what you might call a true psychedelic, as opposed to something like, for example, *Salvia divinorum* that has profound mind-altering affects, but it's a kappa opiate agonist, so it's not a true psychedelic.

The interesting thing about DMT is that when it's orally ingested it's not active, because it's inactivated in the gut by this enzyme we've been hearing so much about, monoamine oxidase (MAO). So in other words, it must be parenterally ingested either by injection or by smoking or in traditional societies as a snuff, and then it's active on its own. But if it's going to be orally active, it has to be rendered orally active by taking it with an MAO inhibitor, which is the basis of ayahuasca pharmacology.

When that happens, the pharmacokinetics of DMT are markedly changed. From Rick Strassman's work with DMT injection at various dose levels, you get a very rapid rise in plasma concentrations and then it falls off, so within 30 minutes you're essentially back to baseline. But if you take DMT with ayahuasca, for example, the half-life is greatly prolonged for some hours because the β-carbolines spread that out. Experientially, under those circumstances it's quite a different experience. Although the definite tryptamine feel—the tryptamine dimension—is there, it's not as intense.

I personally—and a lot of people—feel that the ayahuasca approach to DMT is much more accessible. I think one of the problems with DMT as a therapeutic compound injected parenterally is that it's so rapid that it's hard to come back with much other than a sense of astonishment. You can't really spend enough time in that state to do therapeutic work, if that's the reason that you take it, and I think that's perhaps one of the reasons that as a potential medicine DMT has been neglected. But now that we're learning more about it that may change.

So that's kind of the pharmacokinetic picture of DMT—very rapidly acting and very quickly eliminated from the brain, at least, where it is eliminated within just a few minutes, whereas ayahuasca prolongs that process.

Let's back up a little bit and talk about aromatic amino acids, because DMT originates from tryptophan, and tryptophan is an aromatic amino acid. The other two aromatic amino acids are tyrosine and phenylalanine and these, like all plant products, originate from the process of photosynthesis. The earlier stages, erythrose 4-phosphate, phosphoenolpyruvate, and so on, those are a sort of black box that represents multiple steps on the pathway from photosynthesis, but in the end you end up with tryptophan. Tryptophan is the precursor for all of the indole psychedelics as far as I know.

I foolishly, bravely, maybe a combination of both, chose this topic of trying to make the case that DMT might have an extraterrestrial origin, that it might have actually been seeded into our biosphere, into the genome of Gaia, if you will, at some point by a superbiotechnologically sophisticated civilization. I can thank Anton for throwing down the gauntlet there, and I'm really sorry that I picked it up, because I'm not sure how I'm going to make that case. In fact, I'm not going to make that case, because as I looked into it, it turns out that the TRP operon* is phylogenetically extremely ancient. It's found in the oldest phylum of earthly organisms, the Archaea, which are precursors to the bacteria, and it may have even occurred before the evolution of cells or about the time that life actually became cellular.

Sometimes phylogenists talk about the LUCA, or the Last Unknown Common Ancestor of all life. It's pretty safe to say that tryptophan was in the LUCA, whatever that organism might have been, which is likely some kind of archaic bacteria. So if you look at the phylogenetic tree here, the Proteobacteria and the Archaeobacteria—all things—they had tryptophan. There's very little doubt about it if you look at the genomic evidence. They also had the genes for synthesizing these other aromatic amino acids as well.

If you look at these aromatic amino acids, which are in all organisms, tryptophan is a compound that's one of twenty that goes into proteins, as is tyrosine and phenylalanine. These are universally distributed in earthly life; there's nothing that does not contain these things if they contain proteins—I think most living things do contain proteins—and in nature these compounds give rise to a number of interesting chemical families. For example, phenylalanine and tyrosine give rise to things like the ubiquinones, the plastoquinones, vitamin E, vitamin K, the polyphenolics, flavonoids, coumarins, and lignins. There are also the indoles, which are also derivatives of tryptophan that spawn a really interesting panoply of compounds that are distributed throughout nature and that have many, many different functions. For example, indole acetic acid, which is what you get from tryptophan if you remove the nitrogen instead of the carboxylic acid group, is an auxin in plants, and in some ways, it is for plants what serotonin is for us. It's actually the compound that controls elongation of the root tip and the shoot; it controls movement of the roots and has numerous functions, so it's very important. It's essentially analogous

---

*The TRP operon is one way of describing the gene cluster that is responsible for tryptophan biosynthesis; it is the set of enzymes that catalyze the last two steps in tryptophan biosynthesis.

to a neurotransmitter-like compound, although it's a growth stimulant in plants.

I don't know if any of you are familiar with the author Stephen Harrod Buhner? Lately I've been reading his book called *Plant Intelligence and the Imaginal Realm*—very interesting book, I highly recommend it—in which he talks about the brain of plants, and actually it turns out plants do have a brain. It doesn't look anything like our brain, but the plant's brain is located just behind the root tip and controls the articulation of the plant through the rhizosphere, as well as its formation of connections and associations with other plants, fungi, and organisms that it might interact with in the environment.

So from tryptophan you get indole acetic acid and other plant hormones, and simple indoles like DMT would fall into that class. There are many of them: you get the phenoxazones, which are pigments; you get ommochromes, the insect eye pigments; also actinomycines, indigo, and many, many colored compounds come from our indole derivatives. These aromatic amino acids are distributed throughout nature, they have numerous functions, and they spawn many families of what we sometimes call plant secondary compounds.

It all starts—and really, life on Earth starts—with photosynthesis. And in some ways that's the real miracle. Plants and other organisms that have figured out photosynthesis—a process in nature that existed long before there were actually plants as we think of them, since photosynthesis started with bacteria—have developed light-harvesting pigments. It's a process that the entire community of life depends on. After absorbing cosmic energy from the sun, plants and other photosynthetic organisms wrap it into useful forms, in the form of simple organic compounds; hence, all of life on Earth depends on photosynthesis. Basically everything that does not photosynthesize—everything that is so-called heterotrophic, meaning that it does not make its own food—can be thought of as a kind of parasite.

Photosynthesis is the combination of sunlight, carbon dioxide, and water. In the process of photosynthesis, plants use energy from the sun essentially to ionize water and use the hydrogens from that to reduce carbon. This is very important in maintaining the carbon balance in the ecosphere, because one of the reactants is CO_2. Part of the planetary crisis that we're facing right now is that we're cutting down the forests, and the forests are an enormous sink for carbon dioxide, so this is destabilizing a lot of these homeostatic mechanisms. This is another example of human beings mucking with these cycles and upsetting the feedback mechanisms that James Lovelock talks about that have maintained, more or less within survivable parameters, the conditions for life on Earth for the last 3.8 billion years or so. Now we're actually possibly threatening those cycles.

So from photosynthesis you get initially simple carbohydrates, and then they branch out into many different important biosynthetic areas, such as the amino acids, the aromatic amino acids, the essential oils, the malonyl-CoA metabolites, and so on. These compounds are more or less universal; they are found in pretty much everything and are the molecules of life.

Then there are enormous classes of so-called secondary compounds, which include thousands of different derivatives, like the terpenes, the alkaloids, the nitrogen-containing compounds, the phenolics—there are many, many thousands of variations. And these are sometimes pejoratively called secondary plant compounds. There's nothing secondary about them, but they do not occur universally. They are only found often in specific families of plants and do not have the universal phylogenetic distribution. But plants make them, and plants, or any organism, usually don't waste time making something they don't need. So one thing we know is that the secondary compounds are not essential for life or they'd be in all living things, but they must have a use.

It used to be thought that secondary compounds were either metabolic waste products, things like alkaloids, or perhaps toxins that function in the environment as repellents or as protective compounds. Actually the current picture is a lot more complicated. In some cases they do act as repellents or protective compounds, but they're more involved in symbiosis. It turns out the whole picture of evolution is changing, and the fact of symbiosis is becoming much more prominent than the idea of nature competing. This model doesn't really apply anymore.

The biosphere is much more regulated by alliances and symbiosis. Essentially cooperation and a form of altruism is the language of plants. Plants speak a molecular language; this chemistry is, as Stephen Buhner calls it, the lost language of plants.

Plants use these secondary compounds to mediate relationships with other organisms in their environment. You can think of the environment—the Amazon rain forest, the entire biosphere—in some sense as a chemical ecology. This is signal transduction. Neurophysiologists talk a great deal about the importance of neurotransmitters, hormones, and this sort of thing in the body as signal transduction molecules, but on the global level, *this* [gestures to slide] is essentially signal transduction. So a lot of these compounds you can think of as the neurotransmitters for the Gaian mind, for the Gaian brain. I don't know if you buy into the idea of Gaia, the notion that the Earth—the entire biosphere—is in some sense an organism that is self-regulating by these global feedback mechanisms. This idea was dismissed twenty or thirty years ago when James Lovelock first proposed it, but now it's thought he was correct, and the Gaia model actually does apply much more than was formally thought. And that implies that actually the biosphere—and organisms within the biosphere—have a kind of intelligence.

We suffer from a kind of brain chauvinism. We say, "Well, if it doesn't have a complex nervous system, if it doesn't have a brain, it can't possibly be intelligent, it can't possibly plan and have foresight and act like we do, behave like we do." That picture is totally changing now, because we're beginning to understand that the brain is not necessary to have intelligence; what's necessary is to have neural networks and to have networks of connections and exchanges. You see these everywhere in nature: the rhizosphere of plants, the mycelial networks with which it interacts, the chemical processes that are going on in the canopy of the forest and in the atmosphere, these are all networks of connection. And what arises out of that is something that amounts to intelligence in the sense that it optimizes conditions for the organism. Without using some kind of awkward terminology to avoid using the word *intelligence*, you can't really adequately describe it; so why don't we just call it intelligence? It looks intelligent, right?

At this point people always say, "You're postulating an intelligent designer, and we don't believe in intelligent designers." It's important to point out the designer is nature; there is no designer outside of nature, it's nature itself that is intelligent, it's nature itself that is self-organizing and self-regulating. The reason nature appears to be intelligent is that it actually is. Over billions of years it's figured out how to optimize conditions to make life on Earth possible and enable it to persist.

At some fundamental level, in fact at every level from the submolecular to the supramolecular and probably even the cosmic level, this happens; because nature is self-designed and self-organized in such a way that it makes sense. And that's often why you see these incredibly elegant solutions. Another good example from Stephen Buhner: a tomato plant that is attacked by mites will actually sample the saliva of the mite and will determine not only that it's a mite that is attacking it but also what species of mite it is, and it will call in exactly the predator that feeds on that species of mite. It has a pact: essentially, it will send out a chemical signal to its ally, to its protector. These interactions are extremely fine-tuned in nature and by all rights, by all evidence, you really can't say that this is not intelligent. This is a very elegant, finely tuned kind of process.

So in the context of that—Tony Wright will back me up, hopefully—the evolution of our species, of the primates, is also subject to the influence of this vast panoply, this vast chemical diversity. It's not just the psychoactive molecules, it's all of these things that modulate the immune system, that modulate hormonal systems and all aspects of living organisms. They're all subject to this chemical environment that is on the macro level forming these feedback loops and these symbioses and so on.

Okay, so to return the focus a little bit to the neurochemicals—and again I know that this is trivial stuff for a lot of you but just for the sake of completeness—these aromatic amines that come from the amino acids phenylalanine, tyrosine, and tryptophan by the process of decarboxylation—removal of the acid group from the amino acid part of it—then you get these kinds of compounds that are neuroactive compounds, and they have many roles. The phenylalkylamines have spawned these kinds of classes of neurochemicals, such as dopamine, epinephrine. And the indolylalkylamines—the simple tryptamines in other words—spawned serotonin, DMT, 5-methoxy-DMT, etcetera.

When it comes to tryptophan itself and its conversion into tryptamines, the first step here again begins with the decarboxylation of tryptophan to tryptamine and then from there to dimethyltryptamine by a series of essentially quite trivial enzymatic modifications, again mediated by enzymes that are ancient and universal—they're fundamental enzymes in cellular metabolism in virtually everything. So from tryptamine, which is kind of the primary precursor, by addition of the methyl groups to the nitrogen, N-methyltransferases, you get dimethyltryptamine, the archetypal tryptamine psychedelic. And then from there, again by a fairly trivial series of steps, hydroxylation—again, enzymes that hydroxylate indoles are pretty common—hydroxylate it here, you get bufotenine. If you add a methyl group to the bufotenine then you get 5-methoxy-DMT and if you hydroxylate it in a different place, on the 4 instead of the 5 position of dimethyltryptamine, you get psilocin. So psilocin is essentially an orally bioavailable form of DMT, in a sense. It doesn't need an MAO inhibitor itself, but should you need one, by a process of cyclization these same precursors can give rise to the β-carbolines; so that's just another step on this pathway from tryptophan to this family of neuroactive, and usually psychedelic, tryptamine derivatives.

Conveniently enough, out of the same pathway come the

β-carbolines. These are fairly widespread in nature, and clever indigenous pharmacologists have figured out these combinations; in many cases they don't even have to figure them out; it's often the case that in plants that contain high levels of DMT or related compounds, you also find the β-carbolines, or you'll find them in very closely related species. Some of the Australian *Acacias* are a good example of that; they are notorious for containing high levels of DMT, but many of them contain physiologically active levels of β-carbolines as well. So in that case you can do a one-pot cook; find the right acacia species and you could essentially prepare an ayahuasca that wouldn't require the addition of another β-carboline-containing plant.

As a result of this process, which goes on all over nature, it turns out that DMT and its relatives are widely distributed. They're not uncommon at all. And we find them everywhere: we find them in the higher plants, in many, many species; we find them in the reptiles; in the toads; in fungi; and of course we also find them in the human brain and nervous system. This is the evolutionary consequence of what nature is doing with this tryptophan. It is a remarkable molecule, because it gives rise to all of these things. If you look at the plant kingdom, people say, "Well, we've identified maybe one hundred species of plants that contain DMT or DMT derivatives." That's true, but that's only because we've only looked at about a hundred and fifty or so species of plants.

Actually, I posit here, and I think I can defend the idea, that DMT is much more common in nature than we imagine. There are a number of genera that are known to contain DMT and other derivatives. What's interesting at the genus level is that the chemistry of one species often reflects the chemistry of other species. We know in Australia there's maybe a hundred *Acacias* that we know contain DMT, but there are twelve hundred species of *Acacias*. Chances are half of them, maybe even 75 percent, contain DMT. *Desmodium,* another legume, has three hundred species; *Mimosa* has approximately nineteen hundred species. So there are thousands and thousands and possibly tens of thousands of plants that contain DMT or other derivatives if you look at it from the standpoint of the number of genera. Another species, *Psychotria viridis,* the key admixture plant in ayahuasca pharmacology—there are fourteen hundred species of *Psychotria.* As a genus they do have complex chemistry, but some graduate student should go through and systematically collect all the species of *Psychotria* and run them through the mass spectrophotometer, or the HPLC,* to look for DMT. I bet you'd find a lot of *Psychotria* species that contain DMT. Essentially, the take-home lesson from this is that nature is drenched in DMT.

These are only the genera that have been looked at that make large amounts of DMT. I would venture to say—and I challenge somebody to give me a big grant to confirm or disconfirm this—every plant contains DMT. Probably every plant, but most of them in extremely low levels. We now have the instrumentation to detect picogram levels of DMT. If you just went outside and started grabbing plants and running them through the extractor, my guess is you would find some amount of DMT in every one of these plants.

The point is that it's a very common chemical. It's distributed throughout nature. I guess another subtext point of that is if the authorities want to control DMT, then they've got a big problem on their hands; they just need to give it up, right, because there's no way. DMT is just far too common.

If we look at the indigenous use of DMT-containing plants—the shamanic plants that contain sufficient amounts of DMT to be useful for someone—it's pretty clear that at least in the New World the oldest shamanic plants were basically DMT plants. The source of it was *Anadenanthera colubrina,* a member of the legume family.

We can look to the statues at Tiahuanaco, Bolivia, at 14,000 feet, where I was just a few weeks ago, and there are snuff trays that they have in the museum there. The statues are interesting because you can see them all over Tiahuanaco, with big, dilated eyes. It's not an alien

---

*High pressure liquid chromatography, a laboratory technique used to separate different components of a mixture.

figure, it's a figure that is taking snuff. In one hand he, or it—whatever it is—is holding a vessel that might have contained *chicha* or something like that, an alcoholic beverage. But in the other hand you can see how the fingers are reversed, and it's actually holding a snuff tube or snuffing paraphernalia—at least this is the way this is interpreted. Tiahuanaco is one of the oldest civilizations in Peru, going back to at least 2000 BCE and possibly much older than that. So if you look at the shamanic traditions in the New World, DMT was at the start of them, and really is at the center of them, if you look at the major ones. The snuffs—the different *Anadenanthera* snuffs, *Virola,* ayahuasca of course, *Mimosa*—these are all in different traditions, but they all boil down to delivery systems for DMT in some way.

And then you look at the endogenous DMT chemistry. Again, the same compounds that you find in plants you find in the mammalian nervous system: serotonin, also common in plants; the different DMT derivatives; DMT itself; 5-methoxy-bufotenine and the β-carbolines; and also melatonin, which is not that rare in plants. Melatonin appears to play a role in the regulation of photoperiods and this sort of thing. Another interesting point that Buhner makes that I like: people say, "what is the function of these psychoactives, what do these drug-like molecules do for the plants?" And you can invoke the old protective compound idea, but Buhner makes the point that they have much the same function in plants as they do for us—they are signal transduction mediators; they're essentially neurotransmitters if you will. But they work on the environmental level, on the ecosystem level, so the term neurotransmitter is a bit awkward; maybe signal transduction molecule is a better way to put it?

The molecular target in mammalian nervous systems for true psychedelics are these 5-HT_{2A} receptors, among others. They are members of this large family of receptors known as the GPCR, the G-protein-coupled receptors. There are many kinds of G-protein-coupled receptors. They're not necessarily all neuroreceptors, as some are hormone receptors, but basically as a class they interact with the extracellular molecules such as serotonin, and they act in intracellular signal transduction pathways. These GPCR ligands include all kinds of things: light sensitive compounds, hormone receptors, pheromone receptors, odors, and of course neurotransmitters. One of these GPCR ligand-type receptors, the 5-HT_{2A} receptors, mediates the effects of DMT and many other molecules of this class of what you might loosely characterize as true psychedelics. It's one of about fourteen serotonin receptor subtypes.

Then you've got the pineal gland. It's hard to dismiss, even though we don't totally understand its functions; we know it has to be important. We know enough about it to know that essentially it regulates circadian rhythms, seasonal rhythms, sexual maturation, and all of this type of stuff. Its actions are mediated mostly by melatonin receptors that are located in the suprachiasmatic nucleus in the hypothalamus—kind of the brain's clock—and its modulation of the rhythms through that mechanism is how our sleep cycles are regulated, as well as how our reactions to light and dark are controlled. It also synthesizes DMT, 5-methoxy-DMT, and the simple β-carboline known as pinoline, named after the pineal gland. Pinoline is both a weak MAO inhibitor and a fairly strong 5-HT_{2A} uptake inhibitor. I'm putting this up here as though it's absolutely demonstrated, and I think at this point we can probably safely say it is—these things actually do occur in the pineal gland.

Jace Callaway, my colleague that worked on the ayahuasca project, proposed that these compounds can regulate waking and dreaming cycles and that gradual elevation of plasma levels of DMT during REM sleep modulates the visions. It's a reasonable hypothesis, but nobody has actually demonstrated it. We know Rick Strassman's work, providing fantastic insight into DMT's potential function in major life events such as birth and dying. It's probably involved in the orgasmic response as well, that's a very plausible idea; there are many plausible mechanisms, and what we need is definitive evidence, and that's accumulating. That will come; I think we are all convinced of that, in this room at least. And of course, you all know of the role of the pineal gland, the importance of it in esoteric systems of the third eye and so forth.

So tryptamines have to be important in human neurophysiology, or they wouldn't all be tied up with the pineal. And we have this strong intuition that there's something going on, but what we lack is definitive evidence of the pineal gland's physiological role. It's quite tantalizing, but we don't yet actually know. There's a lot of work left to be done.

That's kind of what we know about DMT from the physiological angle, from the ecological and biosynthetic angle, in plants and so on. The other thing that we know about DMT that we can't really dispute, based on our own subjective experiences of DMT and our own encounters with the phenomenology of it, is that often the DMT experience doesn't really seem to be that culturally dependent—the effects are often more or less independent of cultural context. Cultures will overlay their own interpretations onto it, but the actual experience itself is not so much culture bound.

I think we can all agree that the effects—if you get a solid hit—are astonishing, awe inspiring, and often terrifying. They are a manifestation of what is sometimes called the *mysterium tremendum,* a profound, tremendous mystery that is fascinating. You can't take your eyes off it, but you can't look at it either. The burning bush is a good example, and that's why I put some credence in this notion that the burning bush was probably *Acacia nilotica,* as a reasonable candidate.

There is often a felt presence of nonhuman entities that is interpreted in our cultural context as aliens, perhaps in other contexts as spirits or plant spirits or, who knows, ancestors, many things; but there is definitely a sense of being in the presence of an intelligence that is not you and not human. And these intelligences are not only there, but they are presenting information and they're very concerned that you get it—they're teaching lessons. Often in the DMT state they're very happy to see you because, "Where have you been all this time, and boy, do we have stuff to tell you!" And you know they do, in the few minutes that they have, and you're like, "It's too much to take in." There's this definite feeling that there's a gnosis that they are trying to transmit.

Here's where it gets kind of weird. People see machines or what appear to be machines. Terence [McKenna] made this famous in his characterization of the self-transforming elf machines. It's as apt a description as anything else—they do seem machinelike. It's hard to tell because there's no sense of scale; the things you're looking at might be the size of molecules or they might be the size of ocean liners, there is no way to tell. They have a definite machinelike, sort of science fiction, cast to them. And that's accompanied with a sense of cosmic vastness and a feeling of acceleration, a feeling of moving rapidly, often through a portal or a vortex or a tunnel of some kind. The analogy to the near-death experience is very strong, and alien abductions, and all of these things. It appears to be the closest pharmacological model that we have for these physiological changes we experience during the process of dying that we characterize as the near-death experience. And sometimes we encounter interesting beings—often very beautiful and not threatening but certainly not presenting as anything human. That's the phenomenon.

I want to invoke my dear brother, because the bard says it really better than anyone else [reads slightly abridged text from *Food of the Gods*]:

> Under the influence of DMT, the world becomes an Arabian labyrinth, a palace, a more than possible Martian jewel, vast with motifs that flood the gaping mind with complex and wordless awe. Color and the sense of a reality-unlocking secret nearby pervade the experience. There is a sense of other times, and of one's own infancy, and of wonder, wonder and more wonder. It is an audience with the alien nuncio.
>
> One has the impression of entering into an ecology of souls that lies beyond the portals of what we naively call death. Are they the synesthetic embodiment of ourselves as the Other, or of the Other as ourselves? Are they the elves lost to us since the fading of the magic light of childhood? Here is a *tremendum* barely to be told,

an epiphany beyond our wildest dreams. Here is the realm of that which is stranger than we can suppose. Here is the mystery, alive, unscathed, still as new for us as when our ancestors lived it fifteen thousand summers ago.

The sense of emotional connection is terrifying and intense. The Mysteries revealed are real and if ever fully told will leave no stone upon another in the small world we have gone so ill in.

DMT is not one of our irrational illusions. What we experience in the presence of DMT is real news. It is a nearby dimension—frightening, transformative, and beyond our powers to imagine, and yet to be explored in the usual way.

He didn't get around to suggesting what the "usual way" is, but I guess that's what we're exploring now.

Shout out to my brother Terence. He had the gift, didn't he?

Let's go back to phylogeny for a minute. I was sort of searching around trying to find evidence that DMT was an alien molecule and that it was at some point seeded into the genome of the biosphere by some alien super civilization. I could not find that, because if you look at the phylogeny of tryptophan and the enzymes that modify tryptophan into things like DMT and if you look at the phylogeny of the G-protein–coupled receptors, you find that these things are all phylogenetically quite ancient. The genes for tryptophan biosynthesis have been identified in the oldest phyla of the earthly organisms, the Archaea, as I mentioned before. The genes for the enzymes are similarly ancient—the G-protein–coupled receptors, neurotransmitter receptors, the family of receptors that includes the serotonin receptors—and ultimately arose from one of these several families, the rhodopsin family, and this goes back, if not to the actual origins of life, then to the origins of multicellularity at least.

These things have been in the biosphere since the beginning. They've had their function since the beginning. So if they were seeded into the biosphere by an alien species, they had to get in an early start.

I mean, we may as well say they seeded life onto the planet, and then life unfolded and gave us what we have. And that's possible; I mean, this panspermia idea is not such a crazy idea, because we know that comets have impacted Earth at various times and that they are loaded with organic chemicals, and this may be one explanation for how life originated on this planet. I think that in some ways you don't really need to invoke panspermia, because I think the Earth has plenty of organic complexity and can invent its own life. And that's probably what happened.

So what do we know? We know that DMT is the most mind-shattering psychedelic so far encountered by humans; we know it's a very simple metabolite of tryptophan that's nearly ubiquitous—and I would venture to say it is a universal of nature—it's a component of mammalian physiology; it does many things in the brain; and it is involved in pineal activity. Interestingly enough it's not orally active, so in most cases it's hidden from human experience. Until somebody stumbles on the very simple technology of combining one plant with another—a β-carboline–containing plant with something containing DMT—and then accidentally, or deliberately, it comes out of hiding, and it manifests as you consume that concoction.

And then we have psilocybin, which is a remarkable exception to all this. Psilocybin is an orally active form of DMT that is perfectly suited to mammalian metabolism and requires no technology at all—all you have to do is bend over, pick it up, and eat it, and then the secret will be revealed. So why does nature do that? I don't know. But psilocybin, especially the large mushrooms like *Psilocybe cubensis* that are big, beautiful, and golden, they're obvious as a cluster sticking out of a cow pie, which is where you're going to find them. So early humans could not have not noticed this—I mean you'd have to be blind not to see it—and being a curious species and being a hungry species, our primate ancestors probably sampled psilocybin mushrooms. Early on, really early on. We really have no way to know. But it seems likely.

So what else do we know? Not much. I think in science it's

important to remind ourselves constantly that we don't know very much about the world. We tend to be arrogant sometimes about science, we tend to be smug about how much science has revealed about the nature of the world and the nature of reality, and we often lose sight of the fact that we actually have a very small slice of reality that we can say we understand. We don't even totally understand that. Humility is not a characteristic that you find often in scientists, but I think we need more of it. I think we need to remind ourselves all the time that we're looking at a very fragmented picture of what's going on. Psychedelics are partly the antidote to that; if you take psychedelics regularly they will remind you that you don't know much. At least they certainly do me.

It's pretty clear from the evidence that we've reviewed that DMT is firmly embedded in terrestrial phylogeny. It doesn't have an extraterrestrial origin, so why is this phenomenology of DMT so much like pure science fiction? What's with the machines, and the elves, and the nonhuman entities, and the sense of cosmic spaces? Where's that coming from? Since I can't make the case that DMT is an extraterrestrial messenger molecule—I really can't make that fly based on the limited evidence that we have—so let's think about an alternative hypothesis here.

That is, that *we* are the aliens, and built into the architecture of the human nervous system is a set of receptors sensitive to DMT and other tryptamines that appear to open the doors to an unseen universe teeming with nonhuman life and intelligence. What I'm suggesting here is that DMT is a messenger molecule. It's a signal transduction molecule that works in the biosphere, on the ecological level in the biosphere, but it's not an extraterrestrial messenger; it's a decidedly *terrestrial* messenger molecule. Emanating from the heart-mind of Gaia, it's trying to send us a message as a species. And the message it's trying to send us is, "Wake up, you monkeys! You're wrecking the place!" It's a message from an intelligent nature to the most problematic species to appear in the course of evolution (a double-edged sword, as we will review).

Most of you in this room are probably old enough that you may recognize this iconic image, from possibly the greatest science fiction movie ever made, *2001*. And the interesting thing about this is that the monolith, the concept of a monolith, is that in the movie it fulfills the function of the mysterium tremendum. It is an irresistible force that appears, it's incomprehensible, it's terrifying, it's wholly alien, it's completely other. It appears to come from outside of time or space or anything that we know, and we are fascinated by it and we can't take our eyes off it, and the monolith shows up in human history at critical junctures.

It shows up on the Serengeti Plain—that's where we first see it in the opening of *2001*—and it triggers the birth of cognition. Unfortunately, in the movie the main innovation of the time is depicted as weapons; the ape turns the femur into something to bludgeon people. But it's a tool, that's a step. Then the monolith shows up again two million years later in a crater on the moon, and then again around Jupiter. The role of it, as I see it, is to pivotally influence cognitive evolution, to nudge us along as we evolve toward some unknown purpose. It influences the outcomes in ways that we don't really understand. The thing about the monolith is that it is postulated as something that comes from another civilization.

We don't need to go to Jupiter to find the equivalent of the monolith; the monolith and its equivalent have resided in nature ever since life on Earth started in the form of these plants, particularly the psychedelic mushrooms. These are pan-global mushrooms; they occur throughout the world. They are closely symbiotic to humans, because they are associated—especially the *Psilocybe cubensis*—with the dung of cattle. Cattle became domesticated probably late in our development, but they—ungulates—were around, and these mushrooms would have been encountered. Once this connection was made, I argue that accidental or deliberate encounters with these mushrooms created the cognitive events that triggered neural evolution and the idea of abstraction and the ability to create symbols and to use our hands to manifest those symbols into physical reality—in other words, technology. So this is what I'm postulating: that DMT, psilocybin, and these types of compounds are catalysts for cognitive evolution. This is why they're there; and they're put there not by extraterrestrials but by the biosphere itself, by Gaia, the mother Gaia in all her wisdom to try to get this problematic species to move to the next level of evolutionary development and at the same time not blow the place up.

In other words, nature created this intelligent species that is a very problematic species. It's like inventing the atomic bomb, or nuclear energy, or something like that: you can do things with it that are quite useful, but it's also extremely dangerous. That's kind of what we are, the most promising species for earthly evolution to go to the next level, but we're also the most likely to destroy the whole enterprise. Nature is both brave and maybe foolish to give rise to an entity like us, the problematic primate. Indigenous people have this notion that these plants are teachers, and this is, I think, a valid way to look at it. These plants do teach us things over the course of evolutionary time, and they teach individuals things that they need to know over the course of an individual life.

What do they teach us? Well, for one thing, they teach us symbiosis; that's probably the main lesson. They teach us an appreciation of the interconnected and interdependent nature of everything on Earth, of all living things on Earth. They teach us that we're part of this process and that we are immersed in this web; we're not separate from it. This is something that in the contemporary era we've forgotten. This is a big part of our problem—we think of ourselves as separate from nature, and this way of thinking is something we have to get over.

They also teach us biophilia. Basically on a fundamental level you come out of psychedelic experience with a feeling for the sacredness of all life and a love for life, and that's an important thing to integrate. They teach us animism: the perception that everything is alive and intelligent. And on the global level they teach us pantheism—the notion that the universe itself, the world itself, is alive and intelligent. This is the worldview of most indigenous cultures that use psychedelics, and it becomes the worldview of individuals in our culture that use psychedelics.

These are not hypotheses; these are not suppositions about the way the world is—this is a *direct observation* of the way the world is. And that's partly the lesson—an important lesson—that they teach. Interestingly enough, it's actually closer to the current scientific understanding of the way things work than all these other reductionist and dualist models. Science will support this idea. As I said, there's plenty of evidence to show that plants exhibit intelligence and that the biosphere as a whole acts intelligently and in its own interest; so this is not an unscientific view at all. Science has essentially taken a long time to come back to the view that the indigenous people have always had.

So what else do they teach us? Well, they teach us different ways of thinking; they teach us different ways of perceiving and being; they stimulate wonder and awe; they stimulate ideation and curiosity. Psychedelic experiences are usually beautiful—*usually* beautiful—so they stimulate our aesthetic sense. They open the door to the universe within and make us aware that there *is* a universe within—a dark continent or perhaps a light continent, I don't know, but it's populated with strange beings and strange vistas that were normally not accessible to us.

So they enable the experience: the awareness of the existence of a transcendent reality that is normally closed to us. Apparently it's not part of our normal reality, and it may in fact be beyond death; or we often have the intuition that this transcendent reality is an affirmation of the notion that there is something beyond death.

What else do we learn from these plant teachers? We learn skills, and in a certain sense, we learn curiosity. If we're not already curious about the world, psychedelics will stimulate that curiosity. It does so in indigenous peoples and certainly in us; curiosity is an innate desire to understand things, to ask questions, and curiosity is the engine or the platform on which science exists. Science is essentially a way to satisfy our curiosity about nature, to ask questions of nature in a way that we can actually—within limits—verify. We can get answers back from nature that are meaningful. That's driven by curiosity. I don't know of any good scientist who is not inflamed and informed by curiosity. That's what ultimately drives the human quest for the truth.

Curiosity gives us imagination. It gives us this ability to form mental images of symbolic structures—abstract images that we can then actually instantiate into reality through our creative minds and our creative hands. We can create technologies, artistic artifacts, all of these things. It enables us to conceive symbolic structures that have meaning and that we can then express in an artistic or technological way. It enables us to build models about perception, about the world, and about the way things work, and we have had some discussions here about how we really live in a model reality: it's a reality that our brains synthesize, and we live inside. It's a more or less accurate model, because it allows us to move about and survive in the world, but it's that cognitive ability that lets us build these models. Essentially this is a hallucination that more or less maps to reality accurately enough. We know from physics or other sources that reality doesn't really look like that, but we have to make it make sense in some way, and psychedelics give us the ability to do that.

So what are the evolutionary consequences of this, if any? As I mentioned, we're curious, we're the problem-solving primates, we're the problematic primates, we build models, and we're the most dangerous thing that's appeared in the course of evolution since the whole enterprise began. For the first time there's the actual possibility that we could muck things up so badly that we could actually completely wreck the homeostatic mechanisms that hold the biosphere together and make life on Earth possible. Nature gave rise to us, and she, or it, or whatever, must in some sense have been aware of our destructive potential. I know that these are anthropomorphic terms, but they're not so far out of place. For one thing, the course of biological evolution and the stately pace of biological transformation of species all goes out the window. Evolution is in our hands now, and we will decide how we evolve from now on. We have the technology to reach into our very genomes and the genomes of other organisms.

Evolution is now a commercial enterprise; it's not about natural selection. Human-imposed artificial selection is now the primary driving force in evolution.

We can build, and we have built, technologies that can completely wipe out life on Earth. We have built and we will build technologies that will enable us to escape from Earth. We may build technologies that will enable life on Earth to flourish for billions of years—there's no reason it can't—but we have to get straight about that. What we still lack—and this is a large part of the lessons that psychedelics are trying to teach us—is we have to close this gap between our cleverness and our lack of wisdom. As a species we're extremely clever, but we're not a very wise species, and that's the fatal disjunct from which psychedelics can heal us. That is what I think the plant teachers, with their proliferation on the global stage, are trying to tell us. The environmental crisis on the planet is becoming more and more dire—people are talking about how we have maybe fifty years left, maybe one hundred years left, before Earth is not hospitable toward life—so we'd better get cracking. And I think psychedelics and teacher plants are getting a little desperate, and that's why you see ayahuasca proliferating everywhere along with this consciousness of the importance of these things.

So what does mother want? What does our Gaian mother who's spawned us, and all life on Earth, want?

Well, the answer's all around you if you look at life. What does life do? It grows, it proliferates, it likes to spread around, it nourishes, it nurtures. We look at evolution and we see that any conceivable niche that can be colonized by life is filled with life. It wants to spread. This is what it does. And why should it remain confined to Earth? There's an entire universe out there for it to spread into, and I think that's life's long-term strategy. Gaia in some gestalt wisdom realizes this: no matter whether we save the planet in the next century or not, sooner or later this ecosystem is going to come to an end; and we need to devise an escape hatch and get out of here sooner or later. Gaia's invented us to do that; it has invented this incredibly dangerous tool that properly applied can actually do this. I think that's what it has done, and I think that's what DMT and these other psychedelics are telling us—that's the message.

First thing, we need to wake up to the crisis that we're facing. DMT shows us the future—that's why it's so alien and science fiction–like—it shows us where we're going to be in a century, in five hundred years, in one thousand years, in ten thousand years. And I can't believe that if our species survives we're going to be confined to Earth or even the near solar system. Our destiny is in the stars; this is where we're headed, and in so doing we are fulfilling the destiny that life intended for itself. So if we are smart enough to take these lessons—what the plant teachers have been trying to teach us for five hundred thousand years or more likely much, much longer than that—then we will transform all of life on Earth, and we will certainly transform ourselves. We may be human now, but once we leave the nest we will by necessity have to become something much more than human. In fact we will have to rediscover what we have always been, but we haven't known; and that is infinite, unbounded, and immortal. Thank you.

DISCUSSION OF

Is DMT a Chemical Messenger from an Extraterrestrial Civilization?

DAVID LUKE: Fantastic. That sums it up, I feel like we can all go home now.

DENNIS McKENNA: I don't think so.

LUKE: Well, luckily we do have some time for discussion but only about ten minutes or so.

GRAHAM HANCOCK: Absolutely fascinating. So all of the precursors—I'm not a chemist—all of the enzyme activity goes right back into the Archaea, goes right back into the earliest origins of life?

McKenna: Yes, essentially. I'm certainly not a phylogenist, but I looked at the data. Researchers are able to characterize the genomes in these very ancient strains of bacteria that are very close to the LUCA—the Last Universal Common Ancestor—and the machinery is there. DMT was around hundreds of millions, and even billions, of years before we ever got around.

Hancock: So that raises the question of Mother Nature speaking to this problematic species, because it implies that Mother Nature was aware that the problematic species would eventually emerge; therefore she laid in place the mechanisms to speak to that species right at the origins of life?

McKenna: No, not necessarily. Nature is very talented at taking useful molecules like DMT, or the indoles, or these kinds of molecules and repurposing them. You see this again and again in chemical evolution, where one of these secondary products that might be a repellent for one species is a symbiotic molecule for another species, or an attractant. So these secondary compounds that nature uses to communicate have multiple purposes. DMT was around a billion years ago, four billion years ago, or whenever; it was around, and it probably had other functions in the biosphere.

But then when complex nervous systems began to emerge, it was a handy molecule, it was there, and it was essentially repurposed. Not necessarily that it lost its other functions, but it was roped in for that new purpose, because these organisms are appearing, they're very interesting, they have all this sort of potency, and their evolution could go in many directions. We need, or Gaia needs, a way to direct that process of neural evolution so that it doesn't go off track. And it's a dicey game—I mean it has very nearly gone off track, and well, it's not too late, but I look at it and I don't know. Many people probably have the same feeling that we're in kind of a race and what is going to win out? Is it going to be the destructive—essentially our misunderstanding of our relationship with nature—or are we going to wake up and understand that first of all we're a part of nature and that we're not running the show, actually the plants are running the show. This is what ayahuasca always tells me when I take it. It says, "Remember that you monkeys are not running things."

And also, remember that you don't know anything. That's the other thing: there's no place for arrogance in human evolution. We should be humbled by the intelligence of nature, and we should learn to treat nature better. It's our mother after all; you should be good to your mother. Hopefully we'll learn that lesson, and that's the thing: until there's a global shift in consciousness—and I think that's what the plant teachers are trying to do; that is, to wake us up—all the other things that we might do to save our necks, we're not going to do. There's so much resistance to the very idea that there even is such a thing as climate change. I think that we can put a good deal of blame on the Judeo-Christian tradition, which for at least two thousand years has fostered the idea that we own nature, that we're not part of it, it's just there for us to exploit. And we're busy exploiting it, and we're busy destroying it. So we have to take a more nurturing attitude and realize that we have to bow to our mother and say yes, we'll obey our mother and listen to what she is telling us we need to do through these teacher plants.

These plants have resided in the margins of human society, in these indigenous cultures; but now, ayahuasca and other teaching plants have taken center stage. They've picked up a megaphone, and they're saying, "Hey, monkeys! Wake up!" And they're getting a bit strident about it, with good reason. So that's kind of what I think is going on.

EDE FRECSKA: On the other hand, nature is known for seeding something that has no use until maybe eons later; for example, the gene of language can be found in rodents, just unexpressed. Or Amazonian tribes, they have never seen architecture, but they have the idea of architecture . . .

MCKENNA: They have the idea of architecture, right.

FRECSKA: So for me it appears that something is seeded; for example, the gene of language. You don't have enough cortex, so nature waits until enough cortical mantle grows, and then the gene expresses. And the idea of architecture—you don't have the stratified society to build pyramids—it was just unexpressed. Maybe ayahuasca helps expressing . . .

McKENNA: So maybe this is what happens: the teacher plants enable us. In some sense they're the visualization tool that lets us see the future and the vision of the future—architecture, technology, machinery, all of these things that come up—they are in some sense preexisting in the genome. They would have to be in a certain sense. This compulsion to change things, to create technologies, to invent things . . . all were seeded in the genome. That's the other thing: I'm not sure where all this fits in, but we certainly wouldn't be as dangerous if we didn't have hands; I mean, that's a big part of what makes us dangerous. I'm sure whales are quite intelligent and dolphins are quite intelligent, but they don't have hands so they don't have the ability to impact their environment the way we do. For some reason, we can't stop mucking with things. That's just built into us, and so these teacher plants are teaching us the skill of how to use our imagination, our analytical abilities, and our hands in a way that is conducive to life and nurturing to life rather than destructive to life. Yet we've got this cultural wound happening, this delusion that somehow we rule nature. We have to get over that, I think.

BERNARD CARR: I'm just very intrigued by this question as to whether the ET [extraterrestrial] element is in the past or the future. You started off considering the possibility that actually it preceded humans but then sort of rejected that and ended up with this fascinating idea that it actually is the anticipation of our becoming the future ETs because that's the way to expand. I found that to be an intriguing idea.

McKENNA: That's what I'm saying. Maybe the earthly genome was seeded into the planet and that is the origin of life. But you don't have to postulate that, because I think we know enough about prebiotic evolution and so on that we know if the conditions are right, then it's going to happen. I don't think life is a rare thing in the universe. I think given the right conditions it's an emergent property of life and of chemical complexity—just like consciousness is an emergent property of complex biological systems. So maybe it's true at the beginning and at the end; that's a nice idea: the ETs come along and seed the planet, and then the planet gives rise to a species that becomes the next generation of ETs. I don't know. Rupert, what do you say?

RUPERT SHELDRAKE: I haven't thought very much about ETs, I have to admit. I mean my main interest in what you were saying was the idea that DMT is everywhere. It seems to me unlikely we're the only animal species to have discovered psilocybe mushrooms, so I'm really interested in how other animal species use psychedelics and what effects they have on them. I know they do have effects, because my scientific career began at the age of seventeen when I worked for a multinational drug company in their LSD research laboratory, and we were injecting day-old chicks with LSD, looking for LSD analogues. This was a bioassay: the chicks were put on a table with a glass plate on the table like this, and the ones with LSD looked down and saw the drop and carried straight on, but the others turned back. So the distortions of height and so forth obviously occur to animals, since their brains work very like ours. So questions that intrigue me more than the one of ETs are what sort of trips are other animal species having? I mean it's very unlikely that these things are confined to us, though we might like to think that.

McKENNA: Oh yes, no doubt, there's lots of instances where animals use psychoactive drugs. The thing that's interesting about the serotonergic drugs—the hallucinogens—is that they aren't addicting. There are plenty of animal models showing that if you give an animal a choice to take water with cocaine or morphine, they will go back and back to it, because they like it and it's a reinforcing habit—they get addicted.

But the serotonergics don't really reinforce the desire to repeat the experience.

In fact, as we know from human experience, you kind of have to screw up your courage to keep going back and back to these things. I mean it's fascinating, but you know it doesn't stimulate the pleasure circuits so much. I don't know what it stimulates—call it the curiosity circuits. Many people in this room are quite experienced with ayahuasca and have taken it hundreds if not thousands of times. Each time you kind of have to get your courage up—you've got butterflies in the stomach, you don't want to do it, and it tastes terrible, and yet you always end up going back to the table. Why is this? Is it curiosity that overwhelms the discomfort that you know you're going to have, either physical or psychological or both? I don't know. Curiosity is a strong motivator. And I guess that's what it is.

DAVID LUKE: I think that's part of the reason we're all here, isn't it? We all have this very strong curiosity drive, and we've come to find out—it's the quest for truth. Unfortunately, we're going to have a break to just refresh our minds.

MCKENNA: I apologize for taking too long.

LUKE: No, that was wonderful. Thank you very much, Dennis.

DAY TWO

■ ■ ■ ■ ■

Frameworks for Thinking about DMT

How do we know what we know about DMT? From what perspective are we thinking? What frameworks can we use to think about this mysterious entheogen? In the lectures that follow, we'll gain insights into thinking about DMT entities via Western philosophy, religious studies, biophysics, and from the viewpoint of Amazonian indigenes, filtered through an anthropologist's lens.

You'll hear from the anthropologist Jeremy Narby, a specialist in Amazonian indigenous plant knowledge who introduced the world to the shamanic worldview of the Asháninka people. The philosopher and computer scientist Peter Meyer, who was the first person to systemically study the DMT entity phenomena, will give a philosophical perspective on DMT encounter experiences from the Western viewpoint. Erik Davis, a journalist, scholar, and connoisseur of weird cultural, countercultural, and cult phenomena gives us a view of DMT entities from religious studies. Finally, Ede Frecska, psychiatrist and pharmacologist, and ever curious about the intelligence of all things, rounds out our lectures for this day by fusing biophysics, psychiatry, and esoteric insight into intuitive modes of thinking.

Weaving these talks together you'll discover that there is no monopoly on truth. This intersection of disciplines suggests many ways to interpret the DMT universe, but the ultimate suggestion, perhaps, is that understanding where one another are coming from might be the only way to understand this mysterious realm . . .

CHAPTER 3

Amazonian Perspectives on Invisible Entities

JEREMY NARBY

Yesterday Dennis talked about many interesting things. I like to quibble. I think that dialogue and exchanging points of view is the way to go. One of the things you said yesterday that I would quibble with is that DMT is often independent of cultural context. I know what you mean when you say that: it means that people from different cultures who are naive and uninformed about the experience report very similar experiences, so therefore we think it's independent of cultural context. Well, yes and no. What I'm going to say today is why culture matters.

There are cultures in the Amazon where people have been taking plants, extracts, or snuffs that contain DMT for generations. So they've accumulated knowledge about how to do it and about the entities that they encounter, and this knowledge is then accumulated in their culture. Surely this is one of the things that distinguishes humans from other species—even though one should be suspicious of lists of things that distinguish us from other species. Nevertheless, we are the cultural animals; we are the ones who accumulate knowledge outside of our biology, through our culture. It's given us a tremendous advantage over other species, but that would be another subject.

Anthropologists always argue that culture is important. It's like the way scientists always conclude that more research is needed, because more research *is* always needed. It's almost a tautology, but it remains, let's say, a useful tautology. "Culture matters" is a useful tautology.

Before describing what I think has been established about what Amazonian people think about invisible entities, I'd just like to position myself as an observer, and as an agnostic. And I'd like to say what that means: it means that I know that I don't know about final causes. This is not indifference. We talked about this with David [Luke] yesterday. Sometimes when people talk they say, "I'm agnostic on that," and it kind of means, "I don't want to know about it." No, agnosticism—the way that I view agnostic research—doesn't mean that you're indifferent to something or even that you give up wanting to know and throw in the sponge. It is that you get comfortable with the unknown, and you feel okay about it. So yes, there's a lot of mystery; we're not throwing in the sponge, but we're sitting there comfortably with it.

What's wrong with the unknown? It's not our enemy, we can want to know it, and we can gain knowledge. But as we know, the more we know the more questions that arise too. I think that the agnostic position, at least when it comes to knowledge, is the comfortable and open-minded way of going about things. Amazonian people have the perspectives they have, and I view my job—getting up here—as reporting on and sharing their points of view. I don't think anybody has a monopoly on truth and especially not in these domains. So I'd be happy if you'd like to interrupt me at any point if there is something that I say that isn't clear.

I arrived in the Peruvian Amazon to do fieldwork in 1984, and the fieldwork that I was aiming to do was political and economic. It involved a situation where the World Bank was funding a road into an area that belonged to indigenous people, in this case Asháninka people. The idea back then was that these indigenous people didn't know how to use resources rationally, and confiscating their territories was economically justified. They would take away their lands and put in individuals with a market mentality. They would cut down the trees and set up cattle ranches. This was called development, whereas it was in fact territorial confiscation and deforestation.

The point of my work was to document how indigenous people used their resources and thought about them—to show that they used them rationally and therefore deserved the right to own their lands. So this was politically oriented anthropological research. It was not mystical—I was not investigating shamanism. I was trying to demonstrate that these people were rational rather than anything else.

The Asháninka had a different point of view. Yes, they knew many plants and animals in the forest. In fact, they had names for about half the species in the forest, which is remarkable given that this is the epicenter of world biodiversity. What they said was that plants and animals were animated by entities that they called mothers or fathers or owners and that these entities were normally invisible, but you could see them and communicate with them by drinking ayahuasca or eating tobacco paste. Now just a word about tobacco: this is not the tobacco of industrial cigarettes; this is the original plant that comes from the Amazon, *Nicotiana rustica*. It contains eighteen times more nicotine than the hybrid blond tobacco, and it has none of the chemical additives. These people are making, for example, *ambil* or *ampiri,* which is a concentrated jam. They boil it down to a kind of sticky paste, and they're essentially taking hallucinogenic doses of nicotine. It is a hallucinogenic plant—I must disagree that 5-HT_{2A} receptors make the true hallucinogen, but we can talk about that . . .

DENNIS MCKENNA: "True psychedelics" is a made-up category in a sense, but it is based on pharmacology. So it's not that tobacco or a lot of these other things can't be hallucinogenic; they're just not "true psychedelics." That's a pharmacological statement, all due respect to tobacco, salvia, and all these things that are not true psychedelics.

NARBY: How about "psychedelic"? We could also unpack that word . . .

McKenna: We could unpack that word all day!

Narby: Thank you! It's true. But in terms of "shamanic," if you're an Asháninka person the word for shaman is *sheripiári. Sheri* means *tobacco.* "Person who takes tobacco" is the doctor, the "one who knows," what we call the "shaman." Before ayahuasca, tobacco is the plant you work with, and these invisible entities feed on tobacco. Tobacco is food for them; it gives them fire. This is a notion that comes up in all the ayahuasca-drinking indigenous cultures.

These Asháninka people—once I got over my initial doubts about what they might be talking about, because the point was to try to understand what they thought—talked about invisible entities, mothers, fathers, and owners.

"In your language what do you call them?" I asked.

"Maninkari."

"So what does maninkari mean?"

"It means those who are hidden."

Okay. They are by definition invisible; that's what their name is, "those who are hidden." But you can see them if you drink ayahuasca or eat tobacco paste continuously; that's the idea. The sheripiári or the ayahuasquero entertains a relationship with those who are hidden, through continual ingestion of ayahuasca and tobacco.

Well, they also call these entities *Asháninka,* which is their word for themselves. They say, "These maninkari, they are members of our tribe, Asháninka. And given that there are maninkari animating plants and animals, inside plants and animals, then the plants and animals are also Asháninka and also members of our tribe. White heron is an Asháninka. Small birds are our many brothers, manioc plants are our sisters. The maninkari establish the kinship that we have with all the other species."

There is some difficulty in understanding Amazonian concepts with European words. Anthropologists have tended to call entities such as the maninkari "spirits," but this word comes from the Latin *spiritus* meaning "breath" in reference to the breath of God that supposedly set us apart from all other species, and as such the word is mainly defined as an entirely nonmaterial principle like breath. The *Oxford English Dictionary* gives the definition of spirit as the nonphysical part of the person that is the seat of character and emotion. The nonphysical part of the person. The concept of spirit contains an opposition between the material and the nonmaterial.

Maninkari, it turns out, are not that nonmaterial. They are essential to the organisms that they animate, and when the maninkari leave the organism it dies. Maninkari are the difference between living flesh and meat. They're part and parcel of living organisms. What distinguishes them is not their nonmateriality but their nonvisibility. Those who are hidden—yes, that concept contains a dichotomy, but it is between the visible and the invisible rather than between the material and the nonmaterial. So when you call maninkari "spirits," what you're doing is projecting an opposition between the material and nonmaterial onto them that doesn't exist. The European monotheistic concept of spirit does not do justice to the Amazonian animist concept of maninkari.

Nor are maninkari deities. The word *deity* comes from the Latin *deus,* which itself is derived from the Indo-European root *dei,* or celestial being. The word also refers to *dies,* and "day" refers to the brightness of the sky—"deity" connotes the sky. Maninkari animate terrestrial organisms and parts of the landscape; to call maninkari deities is to make celestial something that is terrestrial.

Going back and forth between cultures is complicated. It's more than a two-step kind of thing because here we are speaking in English about Asháninka concepts. It takes fancy footwork, and it's important to be careful with each word, which is why I welcome you to question any word I use. I think every word should be up for discussion, especially when we go between cultures.

It turns out that all Amazonian cultures have concepts that describe beings analogous to the Asháninka's maninkari—"invisible beings." One commonality is that these people all refer to mothers that animate plants and animals. These are invisible entities, and they can refer to an individual plant, or to a species as a whole, or even to a protector of a local ecosystem. And these entities are normally invisible but with appropriate know-how—usually involving the ingestion of psychoactive plants—it's possible to enter into communication with these entities and to learn from them.

One of the things that I'm arguing is that there is knowledge already established; this is not speculation, this is what has been established by anthropologists who have been into these cultures and spoken with people for decades and then, essentially, brought back their words. When I start speculating I'll let you know. I've told you a little bit about the people that I worked with, but the fact is there are many different indigenous cultures, many other anthropologists have been there, and many books are already written. It would be possible actually to talk all day about it, but here I'm going to take just three more or less recent examples, examples that are not that well known, and look at what they say.

The first involves the Yanomami people, who live more than two thousand kilometers away from the Asháninka in the area of Brazil and Venezuela. There is a remarkable book by Yanomami shaman Davi Kopenawa, written with the help of an anthropologist named Bruce Albert. It's called *The Falling Sky,* and it really is wonderful. So this is not even a book by an anthropologist; it's by a Yanomami shaman. What is interesting is that he also talks about white people. It's not "here are white people talking about Amazonians"; here it's an Amazonian talking about white people. The Yanomami call white people "the people of the merchandise," who are obsessed with their merchandise, and who are willing to poison the earth to produce limitless quantities of merchandise, yet never have enough of it.

Meanwhile, Davi Kopenawa tells us about the invisible *xapiri* spirits and gives us dozens of pages of information about them. So what about them? Well, first of all, to see them you take *yakoana* snuff. This is *Virola elongata,* the tree, which has a bark. Take off the bark and scrape the resin, heat it up a little bit, and turn it into this snuff that you then blow up your companion's nostrils. I don't know if anybody here has, but I myself don't have the experience of *Virola*. I haven't had the opportunity of doing it, but I'm not sure that I'd accept the offer. People who have had the experience describe it as having a shotgun stuck into one's nostril and then having a friend pull the trigger, and . . .

DENNIS MCKENNA: You wouldn't want to do that.

NARBY: What does Davi Kopenawa tell us about these xapiri spirits? They are the true core of living beings; they animate plants and animals. The word means something like "essence" or "life principle." What characterizes these beings is that they are invisible and immortal. They are invisible because they are tiny, like specks, but when you go in close and you see them—with the yakoana powder—you can see that they are like small humans. They animate the nonhuman, but they are themselves humanoid. They are not that incorporeal, in that they have tiny bodies like humans.

The xapiri spirits feed on yakoana powder, but they also like tobacco. This is interesting because the Yanomami do not use tobacco in their shamanic rituals; they use it for pleasure, yet they claim that the invisible xapiri spirits enjoy tobacco and feed on it, and this is a claim that comes up time and again across the Amazon.

When you see the xapiri spirits they arrive dancing and singing. They can't not sing. Their melodies are infinite, and what they bring, first and foremost, is knowledge about healing. What the shamans do is put themselves in the presence of these entities, listen to their songs, and learn them. The way to do this is to diet and prepare the body. So what we would call "going into the DMT space" is difficult; it takes preparation. Then the point is to pay attention to the melodies and to learn them.

Another characteristic of these xapiri spirits is that they are very numerous. They are very numerous because they don't die, and because they are as numerous as the living beings in the forest. Just as there are innumerable plants and innumerable animals, there are innumerable xapiri spirits.

Most xapiri reside in the living beings in the forest, but some come from beyond the sky. Not all xapiri spirits are well-meaning; some are dangerous, like the *warusinari* insect spirits from beyond the sky who come armed with blades and weapons. In fact most xapiri spirits encountered are armed with metallic blades. One of the important characteristics of the xapiri spirits, as the Yanomami see them, is that they are luminous: they are invariably described as shining, blinding, or resplendent; their luminosity is one of their primary characteristics. So we see here that what is normally invisible is abnormally luminous.

Davi Kopenawa is also adamant that these xapiri entities are not spirits. He says, "You call them spirits, but they are other." I don't think he's studied the Latin etymology of the word, but he knows enough to know that the way that his Western interlocutors use the word *spirit* in Portuguese is not exactly what he's talking about. But given that he's an intercultural agent—an Amazonian person who now comes and speaks to Westerners about themselves and about his own culture—he uses the word *spirit* to speak to people because he knows that's what they understand; but he questions the word.

I don't usually read in public, but I think Davi Kopenawa is worth it, because he's pretty clear about the fact that meeting these xapiri entities is difficult. He writes:

> When they arrive they also hurt you and cut up your body. They divide your torso, your lower body, and your head, they sever your tongue and throw it far away for it only speaks ghost talk. They pull out your teeth, considering them dirty and full of cavities. They get rid of your guts, full of residues of game, which disgusts them. Then they replace all that with the images of their own tongues, teeth and entrails. This is how they put us to the test. This is what happened to me and I was truly scared.
>
> These xapiri are really fearsome. They silently drew close to me at the end of their presentation dance. They did not seem threatening yet suddenly I felt their blades violently hitting me. They cut my body in half in a single stroke down the middle of my back. The impact drew

a moan of pain out of me, but that did not stop them. After they had cut me in two, they sliced off my head, then I staggered and collapsed, crying. Every time new xapiri come to you they hit you in the same way, the cutting edge of their metal blades. They start doing it before you can really distinguish their image. Then they start again once you are already stretched out on their mirrors and you see them dancing around you. Yet you must not think that this only takes place when you drink the yakoana for the first time. This happens again later, even when you already own a big spirit house and you have become a great shaman. Each time new spirits come to you, they hurt you as badly. This is why shamans' necks and backs become so painful in the end. These parts of the body are the ones the spirits like to hit, and the suffering they inflict on you is really intense.

A second example that I'd like to give from the anthropological literature comes from the work of a British anthropologist named Peter Gow, in his book *An Amazonian Myth and Its History*, published by Oxford University Press in 2001. In it he tells us about the Piro people in the Peruvian Amazon. The Piro people drink ayahuasca, and they drink ayahuasca to see. And to vomit. They like to vomit because it cleans their body, and they like to see because it allows them to see everything. It allows them to see the people, or powerful beings, inside plants and animals. They say, "When we see a strangler vine, we think it's a tree. But in fact that is a lie. The strangler vine is a person, and when we drink ayahuasca we see it as a person." And this could be a definition of shamanism: it is seeing normally nonhuman or invisible entities as human, it is seeing the people inside other species.

These *kayiglu* beings—these entities that Piro people see inside plants and animals that are like people—what they do is, they sing. That is their characteristic—when you take ayahuasca, you see these powerful entities, they are like people, and they sing. And what the shaman does is listens in to these songs and sings along with them, and by singing with these powerful entities the shaman then attains the subject position of these powerful beings and sees as they do and then knows as they know. The point is to sing with them so as to see like them and having seen like them to then do something about it. And doing something about it often involves healing.

These songs are conceived of as ways of knowing; they are songs of drunkenness, and it means that they can only be understood in drunkenness. They are songs that allow one to navigate the drunkenness, and they are specific to that state. Author Peter Gow notes that the word *drunkenness* is filled in English with negative connotations that *mareacion* in Spanish, or the Piro word, does not contain. Actually French has a word, which is *ivresse,* that has a positive noble quality to it that *drunkenness* does not, unfortunately. English is usually wonderful, but sometimes it just doesn't deliver the goods.

Kayiglu, the word the Piro use to describe these entities, means "one who generates visions," so that's what these beings do, they generate visions and songs. But if they generate visions, then what do they themselves look like? It would seem that they do not have a visual form so much as an aural, or sonic, form. They are made of their knowledge, and they *are* songs. These are beings made of knowledge and song.

The Piro are clear that when you go into this realm, you get contact with these beings. So as anthropologist Jean-Pierre Chaumeil pointed out, first you see, then you know, then you have power. Vision, knowledge, power: these are the ABCs of the shamanic approach and working with ayahuasca. The Piro point out that it is faster and easier to learn sorcery than it is to learn healing. And it's all very well to go into this realm and to meet these powerful beings and to get knowledge from them, but one of the first things that a shaman has to learn is to resist the temptation of entirely identifying with the powerful beings, because they view humans as game animals. So if you start looking at humans with the point of view of being a powerful being, the next thing you know, you attack them. And so it is unthinkable to go into this realm without ethics. The anthropologist Alfred Métraux gave a useful definition of the shaman: it is the person who by profession and in the name of the community entertains an intermittent commerce with the spirits of nature.

Again, the shaman is the person who by profession and *in the name of the community* entertains an intermittent commerce with the spirits of nature. The community is part of the definition of the shaman because the community keeps an eye on the shaman. These invisible entities with whom shamans entertain a relationship are ambiguous—some have healing knowledge, whereas others have destructive knowledge. And it's actually easier and faster to get knowledge that you can use to harm people than it is to heal them, and that's why it is important for the community to keep an eye on the shaman who is necessarily an ambiguous figure. So the shaman needs ethics and also needs an ethics committee. I think that's worth thinking about for people who want to have contact with DMT entities.

Gow is clear about the fact that the Piro themselves are clear that the kayiglu beings with whom they have a relationship are not sky beings; they are overwhelmingly beings that are related to life in the forest, plants, and animals. These are not deities. These are not sky beings.

So the Yanomami had mainly forest beings but a few sky beings, and the Piro who informed Peter Gow in the 1980s and '90s were not dealing with sky beings. It doesn't mean that no Amazonians talk about sky beings; it just means that mainly what we're dealing with here is what some people have called horizontal shamanism. Horizontal shamanism relates to the plants and animals in the ecosystem and makes sense of the incredible forest in which they live.

The third example is drawn from the work of another British anthropologist, Graham Townsley, who worked with the Yaminahua people, and is from an article called "Song Paths" that he published in the French anthropology review *L'Homme,* published in English in 1993. Francis Huxley and I gave a large excerpt of this text in *Shamans Through Time,* which is an anthology that we wrote in Rupert and Jill's basement fifteen years ago.

Yaminahua people drink ayahuasca, which they call *shori,* and communicate in their visions with yoshi beings. Yoshi are invisible, and they animate plants and animals. But they are also multifaceted and ambiguous, and all reports of them underline the fundamental difficulty of knowing them. They are like and not like. They are the same and not the same.

These entities emit songs, and shamans listen to these songs, sing along with them, and learn to communicate with these entities by singing their melodies back to them, but they use words. And the language that they use to sing to these entities is deliberately abstruse and metaphoric; they speak what they call *tsai yoshto yoshto,* meaning "language twisting twisting," or twisted language. Almost nothing in twisted language is called by its usual name. Jaguars are called baskets, anacondas are called hammocks, and fish are called peccaries. In each case there is an obscure but real connection between the two terms. Jaguars are called baskets because certain fibers used to make baskets have patterns similar to the markings of a jaguar. Anacondas are called hammocks because as they hang from trees they sometimes look like hammocks.

Yaminahua shamans say that they use this twisted language to talk to the multifaceted yoshi beings because normal words would crash into them, whereas with twisted words you can go in close but not too close and circle around them and see them clearly. So it's like with a boomerang: you aim it over there to impact over here. You say one thing to mean another; this is how you address yourself to these multifaceted and fundamentally ambiguous beings who have no unitary nature. So here, metaphor is not incorrect naming, it's the only naming possible.

The Amazonian people have a view of reality in which the visible world that we usually see is a world of appearances that hides a more fundamental world that is normally invisible and contains powerful entities.

What I take away from this brief consideration of different cases of Amazonian cultures that somehow use DMT—this is the Western way of phrasing it—is that one could call them DMT cultures, but actually I think they would resist that appellation. I think that just thinking along those lines is a reduction—ayahuasca is more than DMT, it's a cocktail of different molecules. It's pretty clear that the original ayahuasca did not contain DMT and was made essentially from the *Banisteriopsis caapi,* and even the harmalines, the β-carbolines, have hallucinogenic or visionary properties. We could talk about that . . .

McKenna: We can talk about that.

Narby: Good!

Our culture has not been using DMT-containing plants for very long, but we do have a long experience with alcohol. Take the French, for example. They have been drinking wine for a long time, and they have knowledge about how to drink it. There is a *savoir boire,* a "know how to drink." I think that these Amazonian cultures—calling them DMT cultures is too telegraphic—certainly do have a knowledge that we would gain from listening to and learning from them. One of the things that is up front in Amazonian cultures is that it is not just the DMT-containing plants that are worthy of interest but also tobacco, for example, which implies different neurological receptors. So I think that any serious consideration of DMT entities, especially in combination with talk of neurology, should open up to tobacco, nicotine, and nicotinic receptors.

So yes, more research is needed. I think that if we take seriously what Amazonian people are saying about these entities, it becomes clear that first and foremost it has to do with biology: these invisible entities animate living organisms. They're an essential part of the living organism, and they make the difference between living flesh and meat. When you die the maninkari leave the body, and when the maninkari leave the body you die. If we're trying to think about what these entities might correspond to, then I think that the indications are that what they might correspond to is something that is essential in living biology that perhaps we haven't found yet. This brings up the question of what contemporary biology doesn't yet know, and we could talk about that.

McKenna: Might they correspond to the notion of the life force, or the vital force that has now been exorcised out of biology, maybe prematurely? Would that be accurate?

NARBY: The honest straight-up answer to your question would be yes, in my opinion. But we know that the life force is a discredited concept, so I am sort of reluctant to use it; but yes, essentially what French philosopher Henri Bergson and other people were talking about seems to correspond to this. We know that the life force remains mysterious, and it's hard to pin down. That's what these Amazonian people say about these entities—they're hard to pin down. Even talking to them frontally won't do it; you have to use metaphor around them. And I think it's okay to actually recognize that there is unknown in biology and that we don't really know even just what makes a cell tick and how it really works. We can see some of the workings, but it's like there's an invisible pianist—you know the keys that move are related to the music you hear, but who's moving them?

McKENNA: Well, yes. That's it. Life force was exorcized out of biology by reductionists who were quick to dismiss what they couldn't explain. So you know maybe that's premature.

NARBY: Well, now about reductionism; I mean, I believe in reductionism to a certain extent. I think that boiling everything down to one question can be interesting, and I think that looking at the individual parts and how they work is also interesting, so we don't want to throw the molecules out with the bathwater. You know the entire focus of this gathering, on DMT, I think that that focus is a reduction; it really is kind of narrowing it down to this one molecule. I'm happy to be here, and I think it's good for us to be able to have these kinds of discussions—it's a great pleasure to be here and to be able to put this on the table and to exchange with you. Still, I think that those among us who are interested in these entities and the ontology of DMT entities need to question our own vocabularies and our tendency to be reductionist without even realizing it.

McKENNA: It's terminology. "DMT entities" is to reduce the phrase "unseen entities of some kind that manifest in different ways." It's more amorphous than the "DMT entities." What about the LSD entities or the MDMA* entities? You know we now have an entire pantheon of drug-related intelligences?

NARBY: I think it is nonetheless true that with ayahuasca, with DMT, people have a tendency to experience encounters with entities that they don't so much with LSD. I think that experiences of encounters with entities on LSD are rare, and it's often in high-dose territory. One of the reasons LSD is a pseudo-hallucinogen is that most of the time you know you're under the influence of a drug; but we could talk about that.

DISCUSSION OF

Amazonian Perspectives on Invisible Entities

DAVID LUKE: Actually, I think you're right, Jeremy, it's not necessarily about DMT entities per se; it's about the whole psychedelic entity encounter experience, and DMT is merely a hook on which to hang it. I think that there is a tendency to have entity encounters on DMT perhaps more than other substances, although, for instance, my experiences with *Brugmansia* always ended up with entity encounters of some sort. No one substance is necessary—it needn't just be DMT—there are many other paths . . .

DENNIS MCKENNA: You want entities, take *toé* [*Brugmansia*].

LUKE: Quite.

MCKENNA: They'll be crawling all over you.

LUKE: We can definitely think more broadly in those terms. We'll open up for discussion.

ANTON BILTON: Does this notion that the entities act as an animating

---

*3,4-methylenedioxymethamphetamine

life force to individuals, do you think that there's a linkage there to the daemon of Greek thought? Having an associated essence to yourself, that's separate from yourself, but part of yourself?

JEREMY NARBY: Yes I do. And actually, I have had an experience of a daemon—and psilocybin I think enhances this—wherein an intelligent voice spoke to me, and just who is this voice is a mysterious question, but I think it's central to the question.

BILTON: Because I suppose that one assumes that each essence, whether it be plant, bird, animal, or human, has its associated being.

LUKE: It struck me that what you were saying—about how when the body dies, the maninkari leaves and when the maninkari leaves, the body dies—is a very similar concept to the ancient Egyptian concept of the *ka* and the *ba,* which also, I think, has parallels with the tantric system. They talk about Shiva and Shakti, energy and consciousness, and you can't have one without the other: Shiva without Shakti is *shava,* and shava is a corpse. So when Shakti leaves you're left with a corpse—you can't have them separate without death essentially. I think we could find parallels probably in many, many cultures with what they're saying, though not necessarily having the means to see that through the use of these plants. But again there's a danger of language just conflating different cultural worldviews, but I think we could probably learn something from other traditions as well.

NARBY: Definitely.

VIMAL DARPAN: Science and biology has yet to admit the presence of consciousness. As we apprehend these realities in nature—particularly under the influence of substances like ayahuasca that allow us to resonate with those realities and see them—do you think that those sorts of mothers and fathers are like an anthropomorphic projection upon those energies as consciousness? Or do you think they self-exist in the plenum of nature itself as an "other" that we correspond with? So in other words, do you think that that's something separate from us, or do you think it's consciousness as an animating force through nature through which we, also being consciousness, interact with?

NARBY: I think that that's a good question. I think that I don't know, and I'm happy to be able to sit on that position. That said, if I try to think about what it might mean that, for example, tobacco has a mother, then what are these mothers? Well, what the Piro are saying, for example, is that it's about seeing the person *inside* tobacco. So as if tobacco has a personality. Actually that's pretty easy, because tobacco does have a strong personality—tobacco hooks people really fast. I'm not a tobacco person, it turns out. Many of my friends are tobacco people but not me. But yes, tobacco . . . I can sit on an agnostic position and take no position, by saying "I don't believe in any of this necessarily," but the idea that tobacco has a strong personality, well, it's nonmeasurable for the moment. So officially, we can't even talk about it.

But moving into making sense of the world and trying to understand plants not just by considering them as bags of substances but also considering them as actual beings that perceive and communicate, what we now know is that plants can perceive, they can learn, they can remember, they can communicate. Does this mean that plants are persons? What does it mean to be a person? Well, one definition is that if you can learn, you're a person. Snowflakes don't learn. Plants learn. In this sense they can be considered persons. So then the tobacco person, who is this person? I still don't know, I don't know the realm in which she or he lives, but I can feel the personality. Obviously there is something that is there; that is, if you want to reduce it down to . . .

McKenna: Tobacco is not a she.

NARBY: Well, there you go! And that's one of the problems with our vocabulary. Often people are talking about mother ayahuasca; truth is that in half the indigenous cultures of the Amazon ayahuasca is a masculine entity.

McKenna: Jeremy, when you take ayahuasca with the Ashâninka, do you see these hidden beings that they see?

Narby: A few times, and it's true that with toé it kind of turns up the visuals, but I don't recommend toé by any means.

McKenna: Yes, right, but let's leave toé out of it. Toé will give you entities, I think, but I guess my question is when you take the ayahuasca with the Ashâninka, do you see the Ashâninka brand of entities? When you take it with another group or when you take it by yourself, what kind of entities do you see?

Narby: I have had the experience that I described in the first chapter of *The Cosmic Serpent;* this was in 1985. Well, it was a long time ago that it happened. Still, I remember vividly, thirty years ago, seeing enormous fluorescent serpents that started telling me how small and unimportant I was and so on. And yes, this was a Weltanschauung-altering experience. Also, a terrifying experience, and I think that the dose at which I need to take ayahuasca to see these entities is not necessarily a dose that I want to have, or go there, again. So you know it's not, "been there, done that," it's "been there, it's rough, it's mind blowing," and how many times do you need your mind blown? So the ayahuasca experiences that I have tended to go for over the years, to answer your question, is sort of lower dose. And I'm looking for ideas, new points of view, and information about the path I'm on; so I'm not actually looking for deep-water encounters with powerful spirits that cut me to bits and so forth. But you know, if other people want to go there that's fine. I know that that place exists, and I know how to get there. And so do other people.

Luke: Speaking of the Yaminahua, I love the way they use metaphor to talk about or to talk with these beings. You see a similar thing with the Wixarika [the Huicholes]. When they set out on their pilgrimage they change the name of everything: all the nouns get turned on their heads, the road becomes the sky, and so on. But my question is: you said these psychedelically encountered beings are culturally mediated to some extent, so where is the cultural mediation in these different cultural perspectives on these beings? For instance, the Yanomami, who are known as the fierce people—is that right? They are quite warriorlike and fight a lot intertribally and intratribally, so their beings have sharp weapons and cut them to bits. Is this a cultural overlay? Is this culturally mediated, or is this really just an emanation of the beings themselves?

NARBY: My position is that I presuppose that what people are telling me is what they actually think. So in this case, I presuppose that the Amazonian people I was referring to, when they say that they go into this realm and they see these entities and this is what they're like, they're describing their experience just as any DMT-taking person who'd go and have an experience and then would come back and talk about it. It's obviously culturally mediated in the sense that if you're English and you have that experience and you come back and you speak about it in English, then you're going to use certain words. But I think that the experience of this realm does transcend culture to a large extent . . .

McKENNA: So it's *described* through cultural filters.

NARBY: Yes, precisely. If you are part of a culture that doesn't have words for this stuff, then you come back from one of these experiences and you speak gibberish for a while and your friends think you're weird, and then slowly but surely it seeps into the culture. And actually I think yesterday's first presentation was showing how it can seep into the culture in surprising ways. For example, the Yanomami have words for the experience: these are xapiri and this is what we know about them—they sing and bring knowledge about healing; but some of them are nasty, and they're often armed. This is like people who have been to and have explored an unknown territory and have come back with reports from it.

And these different Amazonian cultures that are separated by thousands of kilometers report very similar things about these entities. Then they come back into their own culture and download it, as it were. I think that it's easier to drink ayahuasca if you're a Piro person and you've grown up with people in your family who have had this experience and who've talked about it than if you're just a naive person from London. That's what I meant by cultural mediation.

LUKE: I absolutely agree. So is there a sense that if we could somehow peel back the linguistic bits where there was a mediation through language that gives us cultural overlay, then we would find underneath that there are core experiences that are shared across cultures? The encounter with little beings, for instance, seems quite common—that they emanate light, or that they sing, or that they teach healing—and there seems to be some commonalities beyond the cultural memes that are applied to them by those individual groups.

NARBY: Yes, I think it would be really interesting research. You'd have to be careful, of course, about the language you use. Let's say we're going to do it in English. It would mean being self-critical about English words from the get-go, and every time you use one, like spirit, like deity, even words like nature, all these words need unpacking. It doesn't mean we can't use them or that we have to remain silent, but we've got to be aware of the connotations of our own vocabularies. So then, we do this investigation, in English say, and we read different Amazonian sources— I think it would be interesting to expand this kind of approach to what all the different cultures in the Amazon, including Mestizo cultures, say about these entities—and look for the similarities and differences and then take that and compare it to other traditions again. It would be very interesting to see the commonalities and the differences, depending on the plants used or the plants not used.

McKENNA: Some of those commonalities might extend to the DMT *landscape* as well. We have created a vocabulary around these DMT entities, and we're usually confined to English. Our concepts are not automatically less valid than the other concepts; the Asháninka, the Piro, and the Yanomami also use language, so they filter these experiences through their language, through those limitations. I think we all kind of agree that the phenomenon itself is translinguistic or metalinguistic. It's very hard to apply any kind of language to an accurate description of just what is going on, so we're limited.

NARBY: Well, I thank you for saying that because it's true. It's one of the points I wanted to make or that I think was implicit, which is that clearly for people who are familiar with DMT reports, listening to these Amazonian reports they see these commonalities—like the luminosity, for example. I think that some of Rick Strassman's collaborators or the people who participated came back with the desire to heal, for example. The transformation that some people got out of the experience was their new desire to help other people. This is confirmed in that what these encounters are first and foremost about is getting knowledge from these entities that involves healing.

One thing that the Amazonians report a lot more than DMT users is the importance of singing and learning the songs, and that how you interact with these entities is by paying attention to the sounds that they emit, which is how you learn from them. So maybe that is a suggestion for further research. Then there is this entire question of ethics; one finally does hear quite a bit about ethics from Amazonian people because actually people are uptight about sorcery. Anybody who's putting their head into this reality is going to get knowledge and power and can come back and use it against us. Half of Amazonian shamanism is attack sorcery. This kind of gets hidden when ayahuasca is brought into the West. We don't talk about the kind of shadow side of it, nor do we hear too much about the shadow side in the DMT research and contact with these entities. I deliberately mentioned the *warusinari* insect beings that are from beyond the sky and come at you with their blades and weapons in reference to the praying mantis brain surgeons that DMT users encounter. The Yanomami people confirm that when you use DMT snuff these are the kinds of entities you run into. And it's not easy.

ANDREW GALLIMORE: In Anton [Bilton]'s introduction on Tuesday he said that if you're here, then you should really be open to the idea that mind or consciousness precedes matter. I would say no, there is no need for matter, so to speak. Consciousness is this self-organizing self-complexifying creature that takes many wondrous forms, including this set of forms in this room, but we shouldn't assume that consciousness only takes forms that we can interact with all the time. We wrestle with the idea of the spirit world because we have this horrible creature in our philosophy called matter, which somehow gives rise to consciousness when it's organized in a certain way—that's the problem. Once we get rid of this illusory matter, as the Hindus have been telling us for thousands of years, and realize actually it's just structured consciousness that has this irresistible urge to self-organize and self-complexify and take strange forms including the forms in this room, then it's not surprising when our brain—a kind of a self-complexified structure in consciousness itself—when you change the way that it's writhing and seething by changing the chemistry—starts to tune in, or resonate was the word you used, with creatures from elsewhere within this great grand matrix of mind.

McKenna: I mean, the concept of life force, this classical Victorian concept, was exorcised out of biology probably for good reason. So when I said it was premature maybe I was being a little bit facetious, but it is exactly as you say. These are all consequences of this dualistic perspective, which is very hard to get away from, it seems. Essentially I'm agreeing with you, absolutely; I think that the property of these self-organizing systems—life and other things—you can't even confine it necessarily to biology. You know matter itself, whether animate or inanimate, has this ability to self-organize and manifest these emergent properties, which again sort of goes back to the indigenous perspective on animism. It doesn't stop with biology—in an animistic culture the rocks are alive, everything is alive and intelligent. This isn't that far from Whitehead's idea, which was very much about this: everything is an organism, the electron is an organism, so there is something about matter itself or the processes that give rise to matter that manifest this sort of self-organizing and I dare say even intelligent quality. But you're saying it's not even matter, rather it's precedent to matter?

GALLIMORE: I don't think you need to invoke matter; matter is a process, a process of self-organization, of self-complexification, that consciousness does. So we don't need to invoke this other noumenal world of solid matter, because then we run into all these problems that I've been talking about.

McKENNA: So what you're saying is that we are all, it's all, a dream.

GALLIMORE: It's all consciousness . . .

McKENNA: Something is dreaming it, or consciousness itself?

LUKE: Sorry, I think we've strayed a little bit off topic here, but I think it's very interesting. I think Rupert might weigh in on this.

RUPERT SHELDRAKE: Well, not on this particular philosophical discussion, although it's one I'm very interested in; I'm more interested in a question of fact. So Jeremy . . .

McKENNA: Bothersome fact.

SHELDRAKE: Well, no, just the classification of these entities. You say they are principally biological, so what I was interested in is whether they have categories of entities that are totally disembodied, or whether most of these entities, or all of the entities, they encounter are grounded in plants and animals?

NARBY: Yes, well, that's a key question, and I think it would take looking into it more to be able to answer it properly. What I gather is that these entities can be detached from bodies but most of the time are not. What they mainly do is animate bodies. But then when the bodies die, they leave the bodies. So there seems to be an "ecology of souls," I think is what you quoted Terence as saying? They seem to float around like radio waves, one of my informants told me. So I said, "Where are they?" and he said, "Oh, well, they're in the air, like radio waves, they're all over the place; you don't see them, but they're there, and if you can actually tune into them then you can pick them up."

SHELDRAKE: Do they sometimes tune into the entity of a particular tree or a particular animal or is it the trees, the species in general?

NARBY: Yes, that's the idea, which is that you diet a specific tree. So we actually talk a lot about ayahuasca, but in the Amazonian view of plant medicine, or plant shamanism, there are many plant teachers. The big trees, for example, are serious teachers. The way that you learn from them is you diet them. You refrain from taking certain foods, you maintain sexual abstinence, and then you take an extract of the bark of this tree. You drink a considerable quantity of it over several days and see, for example, how it informs your dreams. And that's how you can learn, and some trees are more knowledgeable and even more dangerous than others.

SHELDRAKE: So that's a specific tree you are drinking?

NARBY: A specific tree.

SHELDRAKE: And you find out this information through drinking an extract of it?

NARBY: That's right.

VIMAL DARPAN: In fact, how the knowledge comes is through the communion with these plant spirits that occupy these trees; you know, lupinitus, chuchi washo, ashpo washi [all phonetic]. Many of them, when you diet them under the circumstances that Jeremy just said, come to speak to you in dreams. This is the way they classically gain information about the plants and find out their ways of usage for healing, as opposed to our way in the West of somehow observing them and looking at them analytically. So it's a difficult thing to verify, but they do give information, very solid information.

ERIK DAVIS: I was kind of processing your earlier question, David [Luke]. You asked a very interesting question, which is what do we say about the differences between commonalities of these entities and their specific differences? It's an interesting problem: if we're going to say that there's some kind of phenomenon, then why is it the case that all these different cultures have slightly different spins on it and what do we do with those differences? And you're like, "Well, is there a way to peel away the specific cultural projection onto this actual phenomenon that we could identify according to the structural principles, or some kind of general principles?" And what I was processing on it is that this is a wonderful example of a fundamental schema that we have in the West about how to organize reality and knowledge. That schema, which is quite challenged by Amazonian ontologies, is that there's nature out there, the world, the objective world that we can understand through science, and then there's a cultural world in here, a world of stories and language and of projections. So the goal of science in that case is, "How can we strip away the language to get at the thing?" Or to say, "There is an experience that we can peel away the language in order to get at."

Okay, that's interesting, but I think if we're really looking at Amazonian ontologies and we're taking them seriously as forms of knowledge, then we have to recognize that they also fundamentally are not in a world where there's a nature out there and a cultural world inside. Jeremy's already given us a clue about that, which is the fact that from their perspective these "other"—these plants and these animals—are persons, even in some cases humans. Now in the West we might say, "Oh, wait, that's too anthropomorphic," or, "That's not the spirit; you don't want the human there," or "We're getting away from humans; we are sick of humans." But what this idea of Amazonian perspectivism is really pointing to is that the person—the human realm, the cultural realm that we share—is what everybody's doing. It's just we have to see it from their perspective to recognize it. So the jaguar is eating the beast, or is drinking manioc beer; or these entities live in homes, they live in structures, and the final twist on that is the desire to get at the nature behind the projection to get away from the fact that from an Amazonian perspective it can only be in relation. It can only be in a relationship of "persons" [including nonhuman and even noncorporeal persons] that this knowledge would be produced.

And we say, "No, no, the person is the projection; we want to get at the thing itself." But that's the point: you're always going to be in relation with that. And what we're doing now in DMT and ayahuasca culture in the West is developing new relations—some well informed, some misinformed, some chaotic, some sublime, and some novel in ways that are perhaps very interesting. But it's just good to always remember—especially, you know, in a room full of scientists, we're all naturalists in that sense—how easy it is to slip into that mode unquestioned, the mode of "there's a world out there and we're projecting onto it" as opposed to "a world that's always in cultural relation."

LUKE: Would you like to come back in, Jeremy?

NARBY: Luis?

LUIS LUNA: I wanted to add that the concept of spirit, soul, or animism is not only plants and animals; it is in everything. I remember once one of my teachers was boiling ayahuasca, and bubbles were coming out. He said, "Look! These are people, the bubbles are people." Or in the river, you have a whirlpool and that's people. Even transient phenomena are spirits or people. And the idea is the perspectivism, as in that for a jaguar, we are the jaguar. For them, they are the people. You know for a child in the jaguar world, they are the people. We are the predators, we are the jaguar. So it's always this kind of shifting perspective.

LUKE: I think, unless you'd like to add anything, we're going to round this one up. Thank you very much, Jeremy.

CHAPTER 4

Concerning the Nature of the DMT Entities and Their Relation to Us

PETER MEYER

Unlike most of the other presenters here, I'm not a well-known researcher or writer, and I have published little on the subject of DMT except for an article twenty-two years ago titled "Apparent Communication with Discarnate Entities Induced by Dimethyltryptamine." It was the first publication to describe in detail contact with apparently intelligent beings in an apparently alternate reality and to speculate on their nature; although, of course, Terence McKenna had already been speaking in public on this subject, and very eloquently, since the early 1980s.

When someone smokes a sufficient dose of DMT, they experience what appears to be a space of some kind that is inhabited by entities that appear to be aware of the observer and appear to wish to communicate something, though what is to be communicated is usually not clear. I term this space containing these entities the "DMT World," because it seems to be a place that can be entered by multiple observers whose reports are more or less consistent with each other and who predominantly report that it appears to them as an alternate reality; that is, something wholly other than our everyday consensus reality.

I suggest that the criterion of real is *intersubjective verifiability*. One or two people claiming to have experienced such entities may be dismissed as hallucinating. But when a couple of hundred people report such an experience, and the reports, while mostly independent, are curiously similar, it is not so easy to dismiss them in this way. And indeed, a couple of hundred people *have* reported contact with these entities, as documented in a page on my website titled "340 DMT Trip Reports." Of those 340 reports, most of which were collected in 2005, exactly two-thirds of them, 226, include references to apparently independently existing entities; that is, beings of some kind existing independently of the observer, just as we assume that material objects and other people exist independently of our observation of them.

Up to now I have used the term "the DMT World" in a phenomenological sense; that is, the DMT World is what most people experience when they smoke DMT. My purpose in this talk is to outline a metaphysical framework for understanding what the DMT entities are, and this clearly goes beyond phenomenology into ontology. Later I shall discuss the DMT World in a more ontological sense.

It is not difficult to observe the inhabitants of the DMT World, since one only has to smoke a sufficient amount of DMT. But reports of these observations currently make no sense to someone who accepts the conventional materialist account of reality, which asserts that reality consists *only* of material objects and their interactions in physical space and time.

Materialism is a close cousin of *physicalism,* the view that only the physical world is real. "Physical world" means the total of, firstly, what we can observe via our senses, in particular sight and touch augmented by the use of instruments such as the microscope and the telescope. Secondly, physicalism says the physical world is objects and processes whose existence we can infer from such observations; for example, genes and molecules.

Clearly the physicalist account of reality is not consistent with the claim that observation of the DMT World is that of an alternate reality in which intelligent entities may be encountered that are not objects within the physical world. Any account of reality that attributes real existence to the DMT World and the entities observed within it thus constitutes a denial that the physicalist account provides a complete understanding of the world we live in.

Furthermore, the physicalist account of reality has no place even for these observations themselves, because these observations are based on conscious awareness, and the physicalist account either has no place for consciousness or supposes it to be something that automatically *emerges* from activity within the brains of humans and possibly other animals. How this emergence occurs, or is even possible, is currently a mystery, and from the physicalists we have only the *assertion* that an explanation will eventually be found.

In the Western philosophical tradition there are three classical questions; namely: "Who are we?" "Where did we come from?" and "Why are we here?" The answers given by the physicalist account are as follows: First, individually, we humans are complex metabolic systems ultimately composed of molecules and atoms that acquire the ability to interact via language with other such metabolic systems to form organized societies. Second, we are the result of hundreds of millions of years of organic evolution resulting from natural selection. And third, this evolution has been driven by natural physical laws, whose origin is unknown, combined with random events, and there is no reason or purpose at all for our being here.

So I wish to provide alternative answers to these three classical philosophical questions, which some people may find more satisfactory than those provided either by physicalism or by one of the organized religions. I shall also suggest an answer to the question, "Can a robot be conscious?" These answers are of a metaphysical nature and are not meant to be asserted dogmatically but rather put forward for your consideration.

First, "who are we?"

We begin with ontology, which is the philosophical study of what is, what exists, or what is "real."

According to the metaphysical view presented here, the fundamental reality is a primordial Awareness, with a capital "A." We can call it "the Primordial Mind" or "God" if you wish. There is nothing beyond or above the Primordial Mind that we can conceptualize. It can, however, be known to some extent by direct experience in what is loosely termed "mystical experience."

There is nothing other than the Primordial Mind, so there are no limitations on it. It is creative but does not create anything exterior to itself. All that exists is from the Primordial Mind. The consciousness of all conscious beings arises from this primordial Awareness.

That consciousness is fundamental was believed by many of the founders of quantum mechanics such as Erwin Schrödinger and Max Planck. Schrödinger is reported as saying: "Consciousness cannot be accounted for in physical terms. For consciousness is absolutely fundamental. It cannot be accounted for in terms of anything else."

Now we delve into history. In the thought of the third-century philosopher Plotinus, the Primordial Mind is called "the One." The Primordial Mind is a unified Mind. In order to enhance its possible experience it created from itself individual spiritual intelligences able to contemplate the divinity of the Primordial Mind and also to form relationships among themselves. Some of these spiritual intelligences are known as archangels and angels. From them, or possibly from the Primordial Mind itself, emanate many other minds. The essential nature of all of these beings is the Primordial Mind itself, since nothing exists that is other than the Primordial Mind.

Origen calls these lesser minds *logika,* meaning "rational natures" or "souls" and has this to say about them, according to the Internet Encyclopedia of Philosophy:

These souls were originally created in close proximity to God, with the intention that they should explore the divine mysteries in a state of endless contemplation. They grew weary of this intense contemplation, however, and lapsed, falling away from God and into an existence on their own terms, apart from the divine presence and the wisdom to be found there. This fall was not, it must be understood, the result of any inherent imperfection in the creatures of God, rather, it was the result of a misuse of the greatest gift of God to His creation, [namely] freedom. . . . Thus departing from God, they came to be clothed in bodies, at first of "a fine ethereal and invisible nature," but later, as souls fell further away from God, their bodies changed "from a fine, ethereal and invisible body to a body of a coarser and more solid state. The purity and subtleness of the body with which a soul is enveloped depends upon the moral development and perfection of the soul to which it is joined. . . . [Origen states that there are] varying degrees of subtleness even among the celestial and spiritual bodies.

We should not understand Origen's talk of bodies in a modern materialist sense; that is, that a body is something of a totally different nature from a mind. This is the basic error that was introduced into modern philosophy by René Descartes in the seventeenth century. Modern philosophy is only now recovering from this basic error.

In his book *On First Principles* Origen says that only the Father, Son, and Holy Ghost are incorporeal; that is, lacking bodies. All "rational natures," that is, souls, have bodies. Among the souls there are angels, humans, and one or more other types of souls that occupy an intermediate position. One of these types of souls is the DMT entities. So the DMT entities, like angels and humans, have bodies. Their bodies are actually visible to anyone who ventures into the DMT World.

William Blake said in his book *The Marriage of Heaven and Hell*: "Man has no Body distinct from his Soul. For that called Body is a portion of Soul discerned by the five senses, the chief inlets of Soul in this age."

This is an important insight and leads to the understanding that for all souls at whatever level, the term "body" can be interpreted as having a dual meaning. First, it is the body as experienced by the soul, and second, it is something not directly known by the soul that is extrinsic to the soul but is still part of the Primordial Mind, which informs the soul's experience.

So the answer to the first classical philosophical question, "Who are we?" is that both we and the DMT entities are among the souls that Origen describes in his cosmology.

We come now to the second question.

Where do we come from?

This question is partially answered by the answer to the first question, since we are souls who have been instantiated by the creative activity of the Primordial Mind or by one of the principles emanating from it. But there is a more specific answer, which concerns our relation to the DMT entities.

In my article "Apparent Communication with Discarnate Entities," I suggest eight possible interpretations of the DMT experience, one of which is:

> The realm to which DMT provides access is the world of the dead. The entities experienced are the souls, or personalities, of the departed, which retain some kind of life and ability to communicate. The realm of dead souls, commonly accepted by cultures and societies other than that of the modern West, is now accessible using DMT.

I elaborated on this idea in a section of my article titled "DMT and the Death State," in which I said:

> Who are we and how did we get here? Clearly we are personalities who develop in connection with our bodies. But are we personalities who have our origin in the development of our bodies?

Or do we originate as hyperspatial entities who become associated with bodies for the purpose of acting in what appears to us as the ordinary world?

I now wish to expand on this idea that we humans originate as hyperspatial entities. Specifically, I suggest that before each of us humans became incarnate organisms in this natural world, we were entities in the DMT World and that during fetal development in the womb we made a transition from the DMT World to this natural world.

A very important article about DMT written in 2012 by Andrew Gallimore is titled "Building Alien Worlds." The concept of *building a world* derives from contemporary neuroscience, most of whose practitioners assume that consciousness is somehow produced by the activity of the brain. One of the foremost exponents of this is the German philosopher Thomas Metzinger. In his book *The Ego Tunnel*, Metzinger speaks of the so-called *neural correlate of consciousness* and defines this as "that set of neurofunctional properties of your brain sufficient to bring about a conscious experience." Brain activity is alleged to "underlie" consciousness, but no philosopher or neuroscientist can explain how consciousness can be generated by what is essentially a system of interconnected biochemical processes occurring in physical space and time.

The orthodox scientific theory of consciousness assumes that a human is an organism existing in physical space and possessing a physical brain, mainly composed of neurons, whose activity is observable and measurable. Such observation *itself* presupposes consciousness, a fact that adherents to the orthodox theory usually ignore. Thomas Metzinger considers the problem of how to explain to us the appearance of a single, unified world to a "self" apparently existing at the present moment in that world. The explanation he gives is, of course, given in terms of brain activity. The brain allegedly constructs a model of a world, a world possessing the qualities of space and time, in which occur multiple objects possessing stable properties. This construction is called "building a world," and when the brain builds a world, then, according to the orthodox theory, consciousness of that world simply *happens*. To believe this requires an act of faith.

This claim, moreover, seems to be reached by a failure to distinguish clearly between *representation* and *appearance*. For example, a navigational device in a car possesses a representation of a world consisting of roads, their geographical relations, rules of the road, and the current position and velocity of the car, but the world so represented does not *appear* to that navigational device. An *appearance* must be an appearance to a conscious being. So when Metzinger attempts to explain the appearance of a world to humans in terms of a complex model constructed by and within the brain, by using the word *appearance* he is covertly inserting the assumption that the world that is built by the brain is a world that appears to a conscious being. Or to put it more succinctly, building a world is not the same as building a *phenomenal* world.

However, the neuroscientific concept of building a world provides us with insight into what a "world" is; namely, it is *the totality of the appearances of a world to a community of conscious beings* (or souls). The consensus world that we believe we live in is the totality of all appearances to humans of a world. Similarly, the DMT World is the totality of all appearances to DMT entities of a world. Obviously, since we are not them, their world is not the same as our world.

Note that we now have a more ontological definition of the DMT World in addition to the phenomenological concept with which we began; namely, the DMT World is the totality of all appearances of a world to the DMT entities.

In his article "Building Alien Worlds," Andrew [Gallimore] discusses the neurotransmitters serotonin and DMT, which are so-called *neuromodulators* in that they alter neural activity in a global manner.

The abstract says, in part:

Arguably the most remarkable property of the human brain is its ability to construct the world that appears to consciousness. The brain is capable of building worlds during waking life, but also [of doing so] in the complete absence of extrinsic sensory data, entirely from intrinsic thalamocortical activity, as during dreaming. . . . [By] regarding this unique molecule [DMT] as equivalent to serotonin . . . DMT's effects may be explained. Serotonin has evolved to hold the brain's thalamocortical system in a state in which the consensus world is built. When serotonin is replaced by DMT, the thalamocortical system shifts into an equivalent state, but one in which an apparently alien world is built.

I believe this idea is a very important contribution to our understanding of the DMT World. However, I suggest that what is stated in the remainder of the abstract, namely, that DMT is "an ancestral neuromodulator," is not correct. In his article Andrew [Gallimore] says:

DMT is an *ancestral neuromodulator*, that is, a neuromodulator that, at some point in our evolutionary past, was secreted in psychedelic concentrations by the brain . . . [but] has subsequently been lost. . . . [In] this ancestral period, the brain would have produced both serotonin and DMT, although probably not at the same time. The evolution of the consensus world-building capabilities of the brain took place under the modulation of serotonin, and was driven by the extrinsic sensory data from the consensus world. However, periodically, the brain was able to switch from primarily serotonin secretion to DMT secretion. . . . [The] thalamocortical system developed an ability to build the "consensus world" when serotonin was present and the "alien world" when DMT was present. . . . [The] brain underwent a parallel neural evolution, in which two entirely separate world-building capabilities were developed.

Andrew is here suggesting that the ability of the brain to build the consensus world and its ability to build the DMT World developed concurrently. He continues:

> Perhaps, however, in order to cement the human species more firmly in the consensus world, the DMT-secreting ability of the brain was gradually lost and only serotonin remained. As a consequence, all knowledge of the other reality was eventually forgotten.

I now give my reason for thinking that this is not correct. According to the received account of organic evolution, new features develop in a species because they increase the chance of survival to reproductive age for members of that species. Clearly the ability of the brain of any mammalian species to build the world it lives in, that is, the world in which it acts, eats, and reproduces, is something that has value both for the individual and for the species. Thus we can understand the evolution of the consensus world–building capabilities of the brain as being driven by extrinsic sensory data from the natural world. Andrew [Gallimore] describes this well in an article published in 2014 titled "DMT and the Topology of Reality," where he says:

> As patterns of sensory data are sampled from the environment, they activate specific column populations and the connections between them are strengthened, whilst others may be weakened. Over time, those patterns of connectivity that are most adaptive to survival (i.e., that generate useful models of the worlds) are selected and the brain gradually develops the ability to generate a stable, predictable and, most importantly, adaptive model of the world.

However, it is not clear why the evolving brain should develop a second and alternate world-building capability. In particular, why would the evolution of a brain capable of building the world of the

DMT entities have survival value for our ancestors? What our ancestors needed was a way to represent the natural world so as to clue them in to opportunities for food and mating and to warn them of dangers, such as an awareness of . . . *large animal with teeth approaching from the left*. Voyagers into the DMT World do not find anything that gives them immediate information about their situation in the natural world, and indeed they may become entirely unaware of their bodies. So it seems doubtful that the ability of the human brain to build the DMT World would have come about as a result of its survival value.

Thus I suggest an alternative view of why this ability exists in the human brain, as I'll now explain. Here I revert to a metaphysical mode, since I am speaking of what has not been established by observation but rather is put forward as part of the metaphysical framework that I am proposing for understanding what the DMT entities are.

I suggest that an intelligent being in the DMT World, which is a "soul" in the sense discussed above in connection with Origen's cosmology, may be born in a human body and that in fact most of us were once souls inhabiting the DMT World who have been incarnated in this way. To examine this idea further we should first consider the development of the brain of the fetus during its time in the womb.

Scientists who have studied this development have discovered an amazingly complex process in which cells of the primitive ectoderm differentiate into cells that migrate and form a pathway for the migration of other cells arriving later that will become neurons. This highly complex process underlies the development of the fetal brain, and sometime in the second trimester the fetal brain has become sufficiently organized and complex for a thalamocortical system to emerge. If Andrew [Gallimore] is to be believed, then at this point the fetal brain is capable of building a world. I suggest that it does so and that the world it builds is the DMT World. I suggest also that the fetus is conscious of this world and remains so for the remainder of its time in the womb and intermittently for some considerable time after birth.

That humans were once conscious beings in the DMT World explains the fact that many voyagers into the DMT World feel a sense of familiarity with it and feel that they have been there before. This also explains why it sometimes appears that the DMT entities are welcoming them back home.

This leads to a problem: the DMT entity is conscious of being in the DMT World. After the second trimester the fetus is conscious of the DMT World also, since that world is built by the thalamocortical system of the fetal brain, presumably with DMT as the neuromodulator. How does this transition of consciousness occur? In other words, when and how does the consciousness of the DMT entity become the consciousness of the fetus?

The answer is that, as said before, DMT entities have bodies just as we humans have bodies, although their bodies are rather different from ours. The brain of the DMT entity builds the DMT World that it experiences just as the brain of the fetus, after birth, will eventually build the consensus reality that it will predominantly experience. The consciousness of the DMT entity becomes the consciousness of the fetus, and eventually of the resulting human, by a transition from world-building in the brain of the DMT entity to world-building in the brain of the fetus. The same world is built in each case, so the transition of the consciousness of the DMT entity to that of the fetus is not a great leap.

According to the view I am suggesting, the ability of the fetal human brain to build the DMT World occurs *before* the ability to build the consensus world. The former occurs before birth, whereas the latter occurs only after birth. During the first year of a baby's life and in response to input from sense organs, serotonin replaces DMT as the dominant neuromodulator and the capability to build the consensus world gradually develops under its influence.

The view I have developed here is, of course, completely contrary to that of those physicalist philosophers who claim, with Thomas Metzinger, that "consciousness is part of the physical universe" and that neural activity of a sufficiently complex sort *automatically* produces consciousness. In his book *The Ego Tunnel* Metzinger writes:

> One way of looking at the Ego Tunnel is as a complex property of the global neural correlate of consciousness . . . [which] is that set of neurofunctional properties in your brain sufficient to bring about a conscious experience.

But neither Metzinger nor any other physicalist philosopher can explain how neural activity can "bring about" a conscious experience. They assume that it just happens and implicitly assume that a *miracle* occurs. They have *no* explanation for this, so they simply adopt this assumption uncritically as an article of faith.

The neuroscientist's knowledge of the brain depends on two things. First, *perception* of the brain and perception of pointers and digital readouts provided by the instruments that neuroscientists use to study brain activity. Second, *thinking* about this information and in particular the formulation of testable hypotheses to make these observations comprehensible in terms of a theory of brain activity. Both this perceiving and this thinking are conscious activities. They do not produce knowledge of the brain as it is in itself but rather allow neuroscientists to construct a detailed *model* of the brain, one that posits, for example, the functioning of a corticothalamic system able to "build a world."

So when a philosopher asks, "What is the relationship between consciousness and neural activity?" he is actually asking what is the relationship between consciousness and an intellectual *model,* in this case, a model of brain activity. But his intellectual model is part of his own consciousness. Those philosophers who assert that consciousness is a product of neural activity are thus claiming that consciousness is a product of something that only came about and which only exists as a *content* of consciousness. Thus they are trying to explain the whole in terms of a part of that whole, which is absurd.

We can now better appreciate the profundity of Blake's aphorism, already quoted: "Man has no Body distinct from his Soul. For that called Body is a portion of Soul discerned by the five senses, the chief inlets of Soul in this age." This is about as clear a statement as you can get that what materialists think of as "the body" is a fictional construct built from experiences provided mainly by our senses of sight, hearing, and touch. There is thus no "mind-body problem" because the problem presupposes a separation between mind and body, whereas in fact body is a part of mind.

However, we can still ask why there are observable *correlations* between consciousness and neural activity. The short answer is that we have no answer, because we don't know what the brain of a human *really* is, just as we don't know what any perceptual object really is. When we see a table we think we know what it is; namely, pieces of wood joined together, with that wood being composed of fibers, themselves consisting of atoms, which consist of subatomic particles.

But as quantum physicists now tell us, when we examine those subatomic particles they disappear into mathematical abstractions. Thus we don't know what a table really is. The natural world as it appears to us is just that, an *appearance,* and currently we have no idea of what it is in itself. And in fact it may not make any sense to ask what it is "in itself." So although we can study brain activity and, as neuroscientists say, "the neural correlates of consciousness," we can never thereby find a *cause* of consciousness.

As is well known, the eighteenth-century German philosopher Immanuel Kant distinguished between the *phenomenal* world, the world of appearances of things, and the *noumenal* world, the world of things-in-themselves. Andrew Gallimore uses this distinction in his article mentioned previously, titled "DMT and the Topology of Reality," where he says:

The only world we can ever experience is the phenomenal world—the world that appears to consciousness. As far as we know, the phenomenal world . . . never reaches out and touches the noumenal world. . . . Consensus reality is very much a functional reality, a phenomenal reality model that the brain has evolved to facilitate its survival in the noumenal world.

I agree with this statement except for the reference to "the noumenal world," where this apparently is meant to be understood as a world somehow "beyond the appearances" and which is equated with the natural world "in itself." However, a world is not something that is independent of observers and in which observers exist. Rather, a world is the set of *appearances* of a world to the observers of that world.

There is no world that is something "beyond the appearances." Whatever it is that informs our senses, which Andrew calls "extrinsic sensory data" and which I suggest derives ultimately from the creative power of the Primordial Mind, is not directly knowable by us. All we can do is to build conceptual models of parts of it. So it is with any world, including the world of the DMT entities, except that they may have a better understanding of this than we have.

Now we come to the next question.

Can a robot be conscious?

This question is very relevant to developments in contemporary society, because some people, especially those who work in the field of robotics, suggest that it is just a matter of a few decades before we have robots who *are* conscious, just as humans are.

Designers of robots that are intended to behave as humans do aim to provide the robot with a model of reality that is, as far as possible, the same as the model of consensus reality that adult humans possess by virtue of the world-building ability of their brains. This model is a model of a world in time and in three-dimensional space, containing enduring objects with spatial relations to each other, one of those objects being the robot itself—or rather the robot's representation of itself within the model.

The robot designers may succeed in this. But this does not mean that such a robot is conscious. Philosophers such as Thomas Metzinger assume that a robot that possesses such a model is somehow *automatically* conscious, an assumption that is entirely unjustified.

As stated above, a human is conscious because at the fetal stage, in the womb, the consciousness of a DMT entity was transferred to the consciousness of the fetus. This transference was made possible by a merging of world building in the brain of the DMT entity with world building in the brain of the fetus, the world in both cases being the same; namely, the DMT World. Humans are conscious beings because the fetal brain acquires the ability to build the DMT World, thus allowing the consciousness of a DMT entity to become the consciousness of the fetus and eventually the consciousness of the human being that develops from that fetus. But robot designers, even if aware of the DMT World, have no way to provide a robot with the ability to build that world. Thus there is no way for the consciousness of a DMT entity to become the consciousness of a robot, so a robot can never be conscious.

However, this does not exclude the possibility that a robot may *appear* to humans to be conscious. Robot designers may well succeed in creating robots that mimic the behavior of humans so well, including their linguistic behavior, that gullible humans will *believe* that those robots are conscious. So before long we may have a society in which most humans believe they interact socially with robots who are conscious, and thus they will naturally accord them the dignity and rights we naturally accord to humans, even though there will be not a trace of consciousness in those robots.

Finally we come to the third classical philosophical question.

Why are we here?

There is a reason for a DMT entity to become incarnate as a

human being, as follows: from the fundamental reality, that is, the Primordial Mind, emanate multiple worlds. Recall that a world is the totality of appearances of a world to a community of souls. The communities of souls that emanate from the Primordial Mind, and thus their worlds, are many and diverse. One among these worlds is the DMT World, and there may be many other worlds. Within them are many souls engaged in activities of which we, at present, know almost nothing. These worlds form a spiritual hierarchy, with greater spiritual awareness being possessed by those individuals inhabiting a world or level of being that is closer to the Primordial Mind.

Many of the beings in these worlds aspire to a higher spiritual awareness. However, an advance to a higher world cannot be made at will—otherwise most of the beings in the lower worlds would already have migrated to the higher worlds. This advance can only be achieved on the basis of merit, that is, worthiness, which is of an ethical and intellectual nature. And the best, and perhaps only, way to attain this merit is to undergo a descent into the natural world in which we humans live and, over the course of several decades of our time, deepen their understanding of the hierarchy of spiritual worlds and—most importantly—acquire a greater moral awareness than that with which they arrived and demonstrate this in their lives and actions toward other humans and toward all living beings.

Thus according to this view there is evil in our world because only in a world where evil exists is it possible to oppose evil and to strive to do good, thereby acquiring or adding to the merit required to qualify for an advance to a higher spiritual world after death.

A similar view was put forward in the second century by Father Irenaeus of the early church as a solution to the so-called "problem of evil." That problem was to explain how a creator of the world who was all-powerful, all-knowing, and all-beneficent could allow evil to exist. Irenaeus taught that God created a world in which humans would be forced to choose between good and evil actions and that only in this way could they mature in a moral sense. A similar but more complex doctrine was taught by his successor Origen, who held, as already mentioned, that God initially created a great number of spiritual intelligences, some of whom, when they grew bored with contemplating the Divine, became souls who were born into our world, which, according to Origen, is one stage in a cosmic process of redemption, in which all the fallen souls will eventually regain their original close proximity to God.

When a human dies, their consciousness is freed from the limited awareness of an incarnate being. If that human was previously an entity in the DMT World prior to incarnation, then, as death approaches, it again becomes conscious of the DMT World. Upon death, its consciousness reverts to the consciousness of that DMT entity but modified by the experiences of a lifetime in this world. That DMT entity may awaken from this life to find itself back where it came from, or if its actions in the earthly life merit advancement it may find itself in a higher world, or if its actions were evil it may find itself in a place of retribution.

The early-twentieth-century anthropologist Walter Evans-Wentz studied Celtic mythology and folklore in Ireland, publishing his findings in 1911 in a book titled *The Fairy-Faith in Celtic Countries*. In my 1993 article on "Apparent Communication with Discarnate Entities" I quoted one of Evans-Wentz's informants, and I'll end this talk by doing so again:

> In whatever country we may be, I believe that we are forever immersed in the spiritual world; but most of us cannot perceive it on account of the unrefined nature of our physical bodies. Through meditation and psychical training one can come to see the spiritual world and its beings. We pass into the spirit realm at death and we come back into the human world at birth; and we continue to reincarnate until we have overcome all earthly desires and mortal

appetites. Then the higher life is open to our consciousness and we cease to be human; we become divine beings.

Thank you.*

DISCUSSION OF
Concerning the Nature of the DMT Entities and Their Relation to Us

ANDREW GALLIMORE: Okay, so first of all you said that one of the weaknesses of this ancestral neuromodulator model of DMT was that this DMT world didn't have an adaptive advantage in terms of reproductive success. It's a sort of Darwinian argument and something I don't really address very well in the paper, so I thank you for bringing that up. However, I would say when you limit this idea of reproductive fitness to the immediate benefits of building a world, like spotting a lion approaching, I agree that's a very acute benefit. But you have to think in longer terms, and I suggest that if the human was interacting with this DMT world, then perhaps information could be imparted—such as the observation of their technologies—that would stimulate a similar kind of behavior in our world over a longer period of time. And you might perhaps think of that as an explanation for why humans raced ahead in the evolutionary game, because of data they received from the DMT world . . .

PETER MEYER: Well, I agree with that. The remarks I made in the paper were based on the standard orthodox evolutionary theory of natural selection, and you're suggesting that there may have been other advantages from being conscious of the DMT world, which are not immediately paid off in terms of eating and mating and so on. I think

*The author has augmented this presentation with additional notes that expand on the topics discussed or mentioned as well as providing citations for the material presented. The revised version may be found at www.serendipity.li/dmt/DMT_entities.htm.

that's a perfectly valid point, and my only defense is that I was speaking from the standard evolutionary perspective.

GALLIMORE: Okay.

DAVID LUKE: Would it be possible to kind of test this, then, through some kind of infusion of DMT and after see how well the DMT volunteers function in the consensus world? Would you be able to go out to the shops and . . .

GALLIMORE: I don't think so, no. No. No. This is my point: you can't restrict yourself to the immediate benefits. Now, I still think that you can explain this. I don't think you need to abandon the Darwinian idea of evolution here, because a creature that is able to build things or use tools in a certain way may be more reproductively successful for various reasons. I mean I don't think you need to assume that just because you're interacting with this alien reality that it has no survival or reproductive advantage—I think you can do that. I don't think we need to abandon Darwin.

MEYER: Okay.

GALLIMORE: But I agree with you. It's an interesting point. However, what you then talk about—this idea of DMT and the embryo—this is something I've been thinking about. Actually when David [Luke] and I coauthored an essay that appears in *Neurotransmissions,* we actually discuss this idea. What I find interesting is that many of the characteristic motifs in the DMT state are often things from childhood: nurseries, fairgrounds, clowns, imps, and jesters, these things. And it could be that in very early life and perhaps in the embryonic stage that you're suggesting, DMT was being secreted and that's why as the DMT levels went down, perhaps they became mixed with images of childhood. I don't know, that could be something, that could be a hint there I think. I think both of our models have the DMT world holding some sort of primacy. You're suggesting that these lower sort of DMT beings come into our world?

MEYER: Well not necessarily lower; I don't say they're lower, but just that they . . .

GALLIMORE: But the idea is they develop in this world and then become a higher DMT being?

MEYER: Well, they may go on to a higher world but not necessarily the DMT world.

GALLIMORE: Okay. I agree with 95 percent of what you're saying; I'll leave it there.

LUKE: I'd like to jump in with an observation as well. This idea about alien encounters, you know some people have suggested there's an overlap between alien abduction experiences and encounters with elves, and classically one of the things that unites both these experiences is that both have these large heads, these almond-shaped eyes. I went to an exhibition of anatomy where they had fetuses in jars at various stages of development, and at certain stages, they look very much like these classic grey aliens. Are these encounters some kind of experiential atavistic throwback to this stage of development in some respects, where people have these encounters with what look, essentially, like fetuses? I don't know where to go with that, but I'm just throwing that out there into the mix. Did you hear that?

MEYER: Not really.

[All laugh.]

LUKE: I don't know if I can repeat it! Okay, so the resemblance of the elves and aliens to . . .

MEYER: Elves and aliens, pointy ears, like Andrew here.

[More laughter.]

EDE FRECSKA: My question is, how can DMT entities materialize in this serotonin consensual reality?

MEYER: Well, the DMT entities have bodies just like we have bodies, but their bodies are in their particular world. I don't say that their brains use DMT as a neuromodulator, it may be completely different than DMT. Maybe they have serotonin as the neuromodulator. But if I understand your question properly, which maybe I don't, the basic point is that the DMT entities are not just appearances or just phenomenological objects in our experience, they themselves have bodies. Because as Origen says, all the souls below the first triad have bodies. And so it's kind of a leap to say, well, yes, they have bodies and they have brains just like we have brains, but why not?

LUKE: I think he's saying that some people, even without the influence of DMT and just in the serotonergic state of mind, will see entities.

MEYER: Some people will see these entities without the influence of DMT? Sure. Presumably whatever one experiences is strongly influenced by the dominant neuromodulator or whatever chemicals are functioning in one's brain at the resonant time. For example, if you do ketamine, you will not see DMT entities, but you may see other kinds of entities in a different world. That world will not be the DMT world; it would be the world of the ketamine entities.

LUKE: Although entities on ketamine are relatively rare, it seems to be, whereas DMT . . .

MEYER: Well, I never actually saw any ketamine entities, but the dolphin man, John Lilly, he claimed to have seen entities under ketamine. But personally I can't vouch for that.

ANTON BILTON: There's a feeling with ketamine of sensing a presence. You don't necessarily see it, but you feel the presence. I'd just like to say, it was a new notion to me that you brought up that I really enjoyed, this notion of us not being visitors to but rather being originally from that DMT world. Because from a personal experience one of the shocks to me was this overwhelming sense of remembering when I first entered that kind of world. It felt like coming home—these were the things, I remembered this, and I've come home. And actually even the greetings sometimes are as if they . . . I don't want to call them relatives, because there was no relative-ancestor thing here, but the persons or entities seemed to sort of say, "Ah, you're back! We're glad you're back. Let's show you this!" So I really like your notion.

GALLIMORE: Is it an alien world or a world from which we have become alienated?

LUKE: Thank you, everyone. Thank you, Peter.

CHAPTER 5

How to Think about Weird Beings

ERIK DAVIS

One of the things I really appreciate about this gathering is something that I also appreciate about psychedelics in general. Indeed, it was probably this reason, as well as personal motives, that led me to spend more and more of my time paying attention to psychedelic studies, going to conferences, and meeting people, and that is the fundamental multidisciplinarity of psychedelics, their multidimensional character. Just in this room we range from science to anthropology to art, cultural theory, personal experience, all of these dimensions. And there's more: the occult, poetry, we can go on and on. All these perspectives have something to say; they all feed into the question of, "What are these things?" and "how are we interacting with them?" That's really my question, particularly from a Western perspective. I'm very interested in indigenous traditions, mystical paths, and traditional religions. But for now I'm most focused on and most interested in what's happening from inside modernity.

One of the challenges when you have a multidisciplinary situation is the trouble of language. Language is difficult enough to deal with even when you're sitting with folks who have been reading the kinds of books you have been reading. It becomes much more difficult when you

118

are crossing between science and art and history. Even the same terms begin to take on different meanings, let alone throwing in something as ineffable and language challenging—if also language inspiring—as extraordinary psychedelic experience.

That said, I like to think of this as something that calls us to an ethics of articulation, which means listening deeply, really trying to understand, and allowing ourselves to be invited into other perspectives. Another thing that multidisciplinarity does is to allow us to see each other's blind spots. Because any discourse, any perspective, any discipline has its own blind spots, sometimes quite strong ones, sometimes ones that are even necessary to continue forward. If you stay within your zone, these will not be exposed, but when we have multiple perspectives we can encourage each other to look at places that perhaps we haven't been looking at at all. From my angle, the history of religions or religious studies—by which I mean the *secular* study of religion, an approach that uses anthropology, psychology, history, literature, and philosophy—has a lot to say to this question of psychedelics. And particularly about the question of entities, this question about weird beings.

As I said, I'm very interested in our contemporary moment, in the ongoing transformation from within the West as we undermine some of the storied axioms that have been driving the West for centuries. I'm very interested in transformations in spirituality in the postwar world, though of course those are taking place against a broader background of the overall descent into disenchantment. One of the things that science does is to develop power and knowledge; in the West these developments literally disenchanted the world. Materialism, naturalism, physicalism—whatever you call it—took a world of poetry, of liminal experiences, and of mythological dimensions and reduced it. This is a classic story we all know. But the thing that interests me is the way in which lines of enchantment continued to run through the Western experience even when that experience was dominated by a scientific materialist perspective. Psychedelics, historically and into today, galvanize these submerged currents that also flow within poetry, within popular culture, within media, and within esotericism and the occult.

There are of course a number of alternative or submerged religious and spiritual traditions that became more visible or entered the West in the nineteenth century, including Buddhism, yoga, hermeticism, magic, and even revivals of Christian mysticism. And all of these spiritual countercultures began to open up to extraordinary experience. Individuals and groups began to develop counter-narratives that challenged the main materialist dogma even as they began to change themselves through these experiences. But there's something particularly potent about psychedelics as a bridge or linkage between science and spirituality or materialism and mysticism. And that potency derives from the fact that, whatever else they are or whatever else they do, psychedelics are material molecules that we metabolize in a physical way that we can understand, at least on some levels, in strictly scientific terms.

Psychedelics therefore play a key role in the constantly fought boundary war between the disenchanted model of the world that is the dominant scientific view and these spiritual counter-narratives that begin to grow and intensify in modernity. Psychedelics open up a space for new kinds of religious experience, for new kinds of mysticism, and for new ways of thinking about God. At the same time these drugs are material molecules that are produced and distributed not unlike other commodities in the market, and we can understand them naturalistically as potent forms of matter. As such, they become a site of this ongoing tension between science and spirituality, or naturalism and mysticism, or materialism and some altered dimension or the world of the sacred. That's why "the spirit molecule" is such a wonderful phrase. It captures your mind right away, and it captures your imagination. Why? Because it's roping together two registers that we generally separate. We usually do not think of spirit in terms of molecules, and we really don't think of molecules in terms of spirituality. Bringing them together, juxtaposing them, fusing them, is an appropriately poetic way of gesturing toward the way that psychedelics mediate these two fundamentally different ways of seeing the world.

Recently I was reading an interview with the neuroscientist Eben Alexander in a New Age magazine. He is, or was, a card-carrying member of the materialist scientific brigade. Then he fell into this coma while suffering from meningitis. Basically he was pretty much gone, according to all of the machines. But during this flat-lined period of time he had an extraordinary experience he identified as a kind of near-death experience.

So Eben had this extraordinary experience, and he came out on the other side saying, "I've seen the light, I've transformed, neuroscience is wrong, consciousness exists independently of matter. In fact we're sort of trapped inside of our meat brains, and when we die we get released again." The religion of his youth returned in his descriptions, and everybody loved it because everybody loves the story about the scientist who finds religion or finds spirituality again. It's always got to be the scientist, of course. With the religious-studies guy or the artist it's like, "Yeah, yeah, come on, whatever, you guys, you're not very rigorous." But if it's a scientist, now we're going to pay attention, even though scientists historically have often been quite religious and quite weird as well.

Eben's story came out and made a big impression and, of course, stirred up some of the all too predictable new atheists. Sam Harris, who's the best of this highly vocal lot, said, "Well, this is all very interesting but really, there's DMT . . ." And then Harris repeats the same story that Graham was telling us, this Strassman-authored DMT meme that's been so widely and surprisingly disseminated. Essentially Harris's skeptical argument is, "DMT is this molecule that floods the brain at the moment of death and produces these extraordinary hallucinations, and therefore we can ignore this claim of consciousness existing outside of matter."

So here we see the phenomenological weirdness of DMT being used as a way to reinscribe materialism, to say once again, "No, no, this is just a molecule, no big deal, it just produces hallucinations, don't worry about it." And at the same time, as we're gathered here to discuss, DMT has also become—especially for people who are otherwise ensconced in a generally materialist view—a major portal for the spirit, for enchantment, for multiple dimensions, and for other ways of thinking about consciousness.

So the example of extraordinary psychedelic experience can be used both ways. It can go both ways. And that paradox, that ambiguity, I think, is one of the key dynamics of psychedelics today. It was interesting to read a bit more deeply into Eben Alexander's account, which also does this weird code switch between a supernatural and a materialist register. Because for him his experience was very literalist. It was what it seemed to be. "I saw heaven and it's going to be good." And if you look at NDEs, they're often having joyful and vaguely Christian encounters. Of course, there is a wide range of experiences, but a lot of people seem to support a particular perspective by denying the sometimes radical differences between the experiences. So Eben has this literalist idea: "What I saw is what's waiting for us."

But look at what he did after the experience, which is of course always the question. We can have these extraordinary experiences, but there is no fixed way to respond to them. We can come out the other side and join a new religion, or we can come out the other side and go "Well, that was weird," and pick up where we were already going. Or we remain somewhere in between, which is where I often find myself, sinking further into ambiguity.

In any case, this is a very important consideration to always keep in mind. However extraordinary one's experiences are, however multidimensional, however seemingly real, they end. And there we are again, maybe changed, maybe not so changed, and once again we have to navigate our way.

In Eben's case, he navigates toward the market. He publishes a bestselling pop book and becomes a kind of guru figure, someone who knows, someone who has methods that he sells people to help them tune in to his vision of immortal consciousness. And then the code switches again. When he describes these methods and this vision, he goes back into neuroscience mode. He says, "Well, okay, so if you have a binaural beat that operates on the thalamus and it produces . . ." Rather than abandon the authority and clarity of scientific descriptions, instead he'll move between these different zones.

And that's the crossroads where we find ourselves in so many ways. We have one foot in a zone of explanation, analysis, laboratory equipment, and the peer-reviewed production of knowledge. This is a zone we cannot and should not let go of. And yet we're also being freed, released, confused, seduced, and marveled into another kind of dimension and another way of being. To stand on both our feet, we need to recognize and operate *within that gap* as a kind of cross-pollinator or oscillating circuit. And that's what the multiple perspectives that contribute to psychedelic discourse should support. It should not just be a scientific conversation, it should not just be a psychological conversation or a conversation about regulation; it also has to be a conversation about the occult, about poetry, about history, and about myth. If we lose the squirrelier side of the conversation, we paradoxically lose our footing.

DENNIS MCKENNA: I just wanted to comment that one of the things that Eben did following his experience was he began to take psychedelics.

DAVIS: That I did not know.

MCKENNA: He's been back to psychedelics a number of times.

DAVIS: That doesn't surprise me very much.

That's why I think the study and history of religions, which is already such an interdisciplinary space, has some really interesting contributions to this discussion. This is particularly true when we consider this question of psychedelic entities, which in some sense is one of the phenomenological elements that are the most unassimilable into the Western framework. You might do yoga and experience oneness or absolute peace with the universe, and you can still square that with what is happening to your endocrine system or bloodflow or proprioception. That's fine. But if you have a conversation with a toad in a velvet jacket, there is not a lot of room to move within a materialist framework, except toward the basket of psychosis or hallucination.

So the question of entities is a strong question, and that's part of the excitement and the audacity of this symposium. It's one thing to study the pharmacology of DMT, and it's another to directly ask the impossible question: could these encounters that people report possibly be real? We might think about this question in terms of quantum physics or science fiction, but in another sense, this is a profoundly *religious* question.

Our very concept of "religion," as moderns, begins when Europe's expanding colonialist Christian civilization starts globalizing. As the West moves around and exploits the globe, it needs to come up with a way of talking about other people's practices and worldviews. So, it comes up with this general category, or it develops a category that already exists. "Religion" is the umbrella concept that is able to generalize about all of these very different kinds of things. And at the center of this is the notion of otherworldly beings, noncorporeal beings, invisible beings, nonhuman beings, ghosts, and myths.

If you look at the various kinds of beings that are covered by this concept of religion, you're going to find a lot of the same figures that people are reporting in psychedelic experiences: elves, goddesses, tricksters, and human-animal hybrids. Clearly there's some real continuity there that somehow we have to understand.

Some people in the community, recognizing the resonances found between different religious traditions and psychedelic experience, point to some secret ancient mystery cult of actual psychedelic use; the fact that the ancestors were tripping explains the similarities of experience. So Christianity is actually a sacred mushroom cult, which is why you get wild things like the Book of Revelation. To me this kind of literalism is very ironic. People go look at a few frescos with mushroom-shaped objects and declare that this indicates a secret tripping society. Or the burning bush is really *Virola,* or whatever.

Of course there was sacred entheogen use in antiquity, and some of these things are real possibilities, even likelihoods in some situations. There's been some interest lately about the role of *Acacia* in Freemasonic rites. So there are some interesting possibilities, a lot of interesting signals, but very little that resembles even vaguely hard evidence.

Besides, however those individual cases pan out, there's still an extraordinary range of experiences of otherworldly beings that we can't trace to underground psychedelic practices. The desire within the psychedelic community to reduce the rich and highly variegated phenomena of religious experience to secret psychoactive cults is, I think, misguided and historically problematic, at least given the associational and fantastic way that most people try to pursue it. The irony is that, to my mind anyway, such literalism actually goes against one of the main features of psychedelic experience and psychedelic cognition, which is that the world, whatever else it is, is profoundly metaphoric. Our experience is not literal; the world is not literal. And yet people want to discover a literal drug at the heart of religious experience to reduce the latter to the former, just like good skeptics. For many I think it is so they don't have to take religion seriously anymore. If it's all just covert psychedelics, then you can just stick with the psychedelics and ignore the other issues that religion and spirituality raise.

For me it seems much more interesting not to collapse these two currents into one another and to stay with this troubling and tantalizing resonance and ambiguity. One way to do that is to reflect a bit on what it means to compare extraordinary experiences in the first place or to compare religion on the one hand with modern, more or less secular psychoactive culture. Comparison is a key category in the study of religion, because of course as soon as you start looking at these things on a global level you notice all these connections, links, and resonances. Indeed, the study of religions in the twentieth century can even be characterized in terms of different ways of drawing, understanding, and interpreting these comparisons. That's why they sometimes call the field comparative religion. How do we both discover and construct connections between Siberians over here and Native Americans over here and Africans over here; how do we draw these lines together and allow them to resonate?

There are two important moments in the development of comparative religion that really have an impact on psychedelic discourse. One of them derives from the Hungarian scholar Mircea Eliade, who was the single most important historian of religion in the twentieth century and who practiced a very rich kind of comparison. His famous and influential work on shamanism is a perfect example. The concept of shaman derives from one particular historical milieu, but in Eliade's hands it achieves a kind of escape velocity. Today many people routinely use the term to cover all sorts of religious specialists. Eliade emphasized the continuity between Siberians over there and Amerindians over here. Some people critique this expanding meaning as too general, as a sign of Eliade's own imagination, but there are good reasons for it. The general concept of shaman functions well in many contexts, so there's a reason to hold on to this comparative category that allows us to talk about the similarities between different cultures, even though there are always some problems introduced by forcing a singular model onto very different historical situations.

Eliade was the ultimate armchair scholar. He read and remembered all the literature and collected and constructed these fascinating connections, putting them together into larger stories that served scholarly, cultural, and modern spiritual ends. This morning we heard from Jeremy Narby about an Amerindian shaman and the visionary creatures that tear these religious specialists apart, chopping off their heads and cutting them up. This is exactly the imagery you find in the lore of many Siberian shamanic groups—beings disassemble the body, then reassemble it with a twist. What could this seemingly cross-cultural phenomenon be referring to? How do we explain that?

This approach to comparative thinking about religious and mystical experience pours directly into psychedelic culture as it starts developing in the postwar period. In fact, before the war, people taking and writing about psychedelics—basically peyote and mescaline—almost never invoked *religious* language. But later people are reading Eliade, they're reading Carl Jung, and they're reading all this stuff in the hopes that there is some aspect of the soul, some aspect of experience, that can *make connections* between our disenchanted, deracinated Western experience and the rich and vibrant spiritual imaginations and lives of other people. Indeed, both Jung and Eliade wrote their books in part to encourage this kind of speculation, this kind of more-than-scholarly discovery—or invention—of a modern mode of spirituality that would discover itself through the mirror of these other cultures.

Nowadays, many historians and scholars of religion have become highly critical of these twentieth-century champions of comparison, and for some good reasons. Some of these reasons have to do with colonialism and with related issues of appropriation and domination. Others have to do with some of the intellectual problems you get into when you impose these singular categories on all of these very different historical and cultural conditions—for many contemporary thinkers, it is *difference* that really matters. Still others criticize folks like Jung and Eliade for being covertly religious thinkers rather than empirical scholars—though the idea that this line is easy to draw has always seemed suspect to me.

Today I think we've gone too far in this critique of rich comparison. But it's crucial to consider some of the problems with the overhasty drawing of comparisons as we proceed to notice similarities between religion and psychedelic experience. And it's also important to recognize how profoundly *difference* operates within psychedelia. For example, anecdotally there seem to be many trip reports that speak of insect beings from another world, entities often described as a kind of praying mantis. Well, the cosmic mantis is not something you're going to find in a standard book of comparative religion. Yet there's something comparative going on, there's a link there, and if you trace this figure the resonances will almost inevitably open up. That's part of the magic and the seduction of comparison.

A more widely discussed sort of comparison concerns the similarity between the abduction experience—whatever that is exactly—and DMT experience. Are these average folks secretly being administered DMT? That seems unlikely. Whatever's happening to them, we have to remain conscious of the way that we are partly constructing these resemblances, these resonances. It's a tricky sort of work, comparison.

It's even a tricky question within the world of drugs. So yes, the phenomenology of the DMT world and the *Salvia divinorum* world are very different. They also work on totally different receptor systems, and it's not at all clear that we can assimilate salvia, or ketamine for that matter, to the category of the "classic" psychedelics. And yet these things are not *so* different. There are often beings, and some of the narratives associated with these beings, to judge from trip reports and phenomenological encounter, are very similar. With salvia, there seem to be different affective qualities—less awe and even more weirdness. And yet there is still that comparative sense of an encounter with beings, with a cosmic or Earth-based intelligence, as well as a harsh brusqueness, a kind of aggression or fear factor that, again, seems very similar.

There are very different things happening in the brain in these cases, so clearly whatever this entity phenomenon is, we're never going to be able to bring it down to 5-HT_{2A} receptors. Even if we want to have a strictly materialist understanding of what's going on, the entity phenomenon is something else, it's some other kind of network effect of neurons and consciousness. To understand that something else, or even just to approach it, we must enter this tricky zone of comparison. And from within that zone I want to suggest that it's vital that we remain conscious of both the power and the seductive appeal of the sorts of robust comparisons we find in an Eliade or a Jung and especially with Jung's idea of the collective unconscious. Jung was a fascinating thinker, but the collective unconscious is not that helpful an idea in a lot of circumstances, at least in the way that a lot of people apply it. In fact, its very persistence within certain communities—while almost everyone else has abandoned it—should tell us something. More importantly, if you hold on to it too strongly you miss a lot of things, especially things about *difference*. Sometimes we may still invoke these grand synthetic concepts, but I think we must be critical and self-aware of the comparisons that we're making, even as we have no choice but to make them.

The issue of comparison, in religion and psychedelics, reminds me of a wonderful story that the anthropologist Michael Harner tells at the beginning of *The Way of the Shaman*. It's a story about the first time he took ayahausca as a young anthropologist in the Amazon. One of his many hair-raising encounters was with these tall dragons with large wings. They tell him that they came from the depths of space and now rule this entire realm. He's kind of freaked out by this; it's the early sixties, and there's very little literature on this stuff, so he doesn't know much about the aya zone. He describes his experiences to some missionaries, and of course they say, "Ah, see, those dragons are the fallen angels, the wings and everything; it fits right in, it's super Luciferian." Whatever you think about Christianity, you can see why you might construct that comparison from that perspective and worldview. And then Harner goes and he talks to a shaman—I'm kind of compressing the story a little bit—but he tells the story to an old shaman. Now there isn't a word for dragon, so he calls the creatures bats. But the shaman seems to know exactly what he's talking about. He tells the shaman they declared themselves the lords of the realm. "Oh yeah, they are always saying that," the shaman says, "but they're just masters of the outer darkness," which freaks Harner out even more, because he didn't tell the guy that they said that they came from the depths of space.

This is a beautiful story about comparison. Harner sees entities he identifies as dragons. The missionaries see the dragons as devils. Then Harner translates the dragons into bats—compares them—but the shaman recognizes what he saw as familiar ayahuasca characters. If you go with the comparison—and why not—it suggests that there's some kind of collective resonance, or morphic field, or whatever we want to call it; there's some kind of collective cultural-ontological framework that creates a consistency to this kind of entity, and yet it gets organized in very different ways.

The other thing I like about this story is its portrayal of a certain kind of shamanic skepticism. I use that word quite consciously, because one of my projects is to trace, articulate, and even celebrate aspects of our supposedly disenchanted scientific worldview as we move into these other dimensions. And this worldview includes a kind of working skepticism. It implies a resistance to giving over your belief, a resistance in some ways to religion in a certain sense, a kind of active agnosticism. Part of my current project traces how secular, rational people, by using medicines or because of their own crazy experiences, move back toward the fullness of religious experience but in a different way. There are very different ways to access and frame visionary experience, but a lot of the pathologies of contemporary psychedelic culture involve not learning that lesson, not holding on to our particular magic, which in a way is a kind of mental magic, a kind of rational magic, that, in the right context and without becoming the master, is incredibly helpful.

I read a quote from Terence McKenna recently. At some point he asked the mushroom, "Why me, why am I getting this whole thing I gotta do?" And the mushroom said, "Because you haven't given your belief away." Now Terence certainly got caught up in his own wild belief system, but he also maintained a skeptical temperament around a lot of the New Age and mystical ideas that crop up around these things in the modern world. There's something about that rational refusal, or hesitancy, I find very noble and very spiritual in its own way. As we leave the world of disenchantment to plunge back into radical enchantment, there is a tendency among many to give up that rational edge and release the burden of skepticism. I don't think that is necessarily helpful, but even more, I don't think giving over your belief is the most integrated and spiritual way to process these experiences. For me, both meditation and psychedelics, as paths of self-exploration or spiritual exploration, are equally about enchantment and disenchantment.

An element of skepticism is also part of the anthropological, indigenous situation. The shaman in Harner's story hasn't given his belief over either. The traditional shamanic perspective, if I can speak of such a thing, is ambiguous. There's a lot of dodgy characters, so you make alliances. You're not really sure who's wearing a mask. "Is this masked? Is it not masked?" This is the kind of questioning that you also find in the Western occult tradition, where magicians engage in conversation with incorporeal beings. You don't just straight up say, "Oh, okay, you're the angel of the ninth heaven, great!" You've got to test it. You're not really sure who this being is because it's a swirly realm. As Jeremy was talking about this morning, these things are both there and not there; they're the same and they're different, at the same time. They *flicker*.

One of the core issues of comparative religion that's related to all this is the question of religious experience. There's a lot that could be said about this question over the last one hundred years or so, and we find a similar kind of approach as we did with the comparative approaches of Jung or Eliade. For example, early on there was a strong emphasis on what we call perennialism, which is the idea that beneath all of their differences, all the world's religions are actually pointing at the same truth, the same experience, the same dimension of reality or the self. They're just different ways of getting to the same place. These ideas became enormously attractive to seekers and psychonauts and continue to help organize how people see these ambiguous things and how they do their practice.

But if you look at the nitty gritty of religious experiences, you also find that there's quite an extraordinary range of differences. So you have to start thinking about these differences. Why is there a whole vein of mysticism that's about encountering a supreme being? Many mystics describe a loving being and say that spirituality is ultimately about some kind of relationship to a loving being. In these traditions, this seems to be the supreme experience. And yet in other traditions, there is no supreme being in those intersubjective terms. There's oneness maybe, there's nature, there's the cosmos, there's the Self; but there is also a sort of absence of a personhood, of personality. How do we reconcile these two fundamentally different views under one perennialist rubric? Is one tradition higher than the other? No, I don't think so. I think we have to recognize that there's a multiplicity of ways to move through this space—there's not one mountaintop, there are multiple mountains, and we build the path as we walk them.

So how do we explain these differences once we acknowledge they are real and that they are not just different interpretations of the same experience? One of the things you have to do is acknowledge how much people—growing up in a culture with its own models and maps and expectations—set up and shape the kinds of experiences that they have. There's a tendency, very understandable, to say, "Well, there are the experiences in themselves, and then there are the ways we narrate them or our projections onto the experience." But perhaps the reality is a little trickier, and the experiences themselves are already shaped and built partly according to local conditions. They're shaped by our evolutionary heritage—by the ways our own minds and personal temperaments operate and by our own personalities—but also by our own cultural orientations and memory banks. If you're growing up in a Jewish culture, you go into a certain kind of experience, and you're more likely to see things a certain way.

So there is a constructed aspect to these experiences. It's not just like there's some pure visionary world out there that we suddenly have access to and that we need to interpret correctly. It's that we are always in the midst of this cultural, anthropological process—individually, culturally, collectively—of constructing these encounters. At the same time—and this is the paradox, the mystery, if you will—these encounters appear to be more than our own construction. There is a visionary remainder and "Other" in the picture. Strict social constructionists will say, "Oh, it's all just fabrication," and I'm not talking about that. What I'm saying is that we have to really reflect and recognize how much of our own individual and collective assumptions, expectations, stories, and so forth construct the *experiential interfaces* with forces, domains, and even intelligences that are not reducible to our control or our expectations. You keep the door open, but you never really know who is walking through the door, if it's a reflection or not. And sometimes, nonetheless, experience becomes *encounter*. There are encounters that irrevocably transform you.

What's the core lesson of psychedelic practice, the lesson that still holds strong after being famously put forward by Leary's research in 1963 and 1964? Set and setting. Set and setting. There's no way we're getting around set and setting.

Nick Sand has two essays about DMT that he published pseudonymously in *The Entheogen Review*. He's done DMT thousands of times, and he's a very interesting character, which really comes through. He offers a mixture of psychedelic antiauthoritarianism and spirituality in his descriptions of his experiences. The article itself was motivated by reading an early chapter from Strassman's book. It annoyed him, because he was reading these accounts about alien doctors doing probes and all of these abduction scenarios, and he was like, "Look, this is just because you're doing this in a lab, you have doctors around, there's a hidden agenda, and so this is kind of ridiculous." His argument was basically that the *setting* was all wrong and that participants were in some sense setting themselves up for a *bad construction*. Instead, Nick argues, we should be in temples, we should have incense, and we should have sound.

But the question of construction does not go away. It's not like it's only a construction when it's bad, like a bad trip is bad because the setting is wrong, but good trips are true and real. If set and setting are partly composing the thing, then when you set up a holier space, that's also making the thing. Not all of it, maybe, but a lot of it. So the sacred emerges not because it's all holy coming down on us. It's that through our art and intention we are building the holy space, building the sacred context, and setting ourselves up for meaning.

I've been talking, again, about how to talk about weird beings, and I just want to say a few more things. One of the problems when we try to bring our modern, science-shaped mind together with this other world—let's call it the spiritual world—is that there are certain habits of thought that go along with the sciences that we bring along almost unconsciously with us as we go into this other domain. One habit is a kind of literalism, a reductive drive toward finding a singular explanatory key. This is tied up with a very dualistic sense of ontology, of what's real versus what's not real. From a basic scientific perspective, we might say that nature is real, and the material universe is what's really real. And then there are our minds, which are projecting onto this landscape and creating cultural stories about these natural facts. Then we bring this perspective, this ontological template, into these other dimensions. We bring these habits of literalizing and dividing experiences into real and false with us as we think about radical visionary experience because we're carrying over these unconscious habits from scientific culture.

I want to suggest a different perspective. It's rooted in what you might call a kind of existential or ontological pluralism. On some level, all I really know is my experience, and all I see is different ways of being, fundamentally different ways of being that share and interface in this messy multiplicity before me. I don't see the place where they all fit together; I don't see the place where there's only one kind of way *to be*. Take fictional characters, for example. We all know who Sherlock Holmes is; there's a certain consistency to him that almost veers into the real. In fact, part of the consistency of the character is that people— fans, writers, and gamers—play a game with his reality. H. P. Lovecraft fans will also know what I'm talking about in terms of this metafictional play with reality. Fictions have a certain consistency to them, and so do values, like valor. Is valor real or is it just another example of a social construction? Either way, valor has a certain consistency to it. It's not real like the table, but it's real in a way that makes a difference. Human laws are another example of how human constructions become more than merely social constructions. Obviously laws are a human creation; we're making them up through purely human processes such as arguments, politics, lies, hidden agendas, and so on. And yet when a law passes, that law becomes real in a certain way and gains its own sort of consistency. In the words of Bruno Latour, we allow it its own ontological pasture.

Rather than just grant degrees of reality to these different constructions—laws are more real than fictions but less real than molecules—we might also just grant that there are different *modes of being*. There are different ways that things flicker into being.

So what can we say about these weird beings, what's specific to them? What is the ontological character, their mode of being? Usually we think either they must be real, at least in some metaphysical sense, or they must be a psychological projection, or a social construction. But there's something else going on right beneath our noses. In fact, I say that if we're wrangling about whether these entities are real or are simply projections, we've already lost. We have already landed on a well-drawn battlefield where all the moves are already anticipated. So how can we sneak up on the issue or move in a different way? It's a big question, but one way that I like to think about it is that these visionary entities *flicker*. They flicker. They're there, and they're not there.

They're veiled. They appear and then disappear both visually and ontologically. That feeling of "do you see it, do you not" seems to be intrinsic to that realm. That's one of the reasons I believe that figures of tricksters and clowns seem so significant here. Not because the whole carnival of entities can be reduced to tricksters and clowns—there's obviously a wide range of beings and manners of presentation. There is something about the space itself that has this character of "do you see it or do you not." Like some shamanic performances, it includes a kind of trick, a kind of prestidigitation.

If the notion of flickering seems a bit too ambiguous, you can also approach this ontological question in a more biological way. Putting aside all this weirdness for a moment, what is one of the most definite things we can say about that person hitting 60 milligrams of DMT on the glass pipe? Well, probably that they'll be back in half an hour or so. These experiences have a more or less definite metabolic envelope. Whatever these beings are—and again, I am not sure that is the best way to set up the question—we also have to acknowledge that their appearances emerge within that metabolic envelope. The question of the reality of psychedelic states, and with that psychedelic entities, is so intimately bound up with biological processes that we might refer to the entire question as one of *metabolic ontology*. This idea helps us place the weird flicker of these entities within the context of our bodies and our almost absolute embedding within biophysical processes. That's just the beginning of an entire line of thought, but I want to leave that there for now.

What I have tried to perform in this admittedly loose talk is not some philosophical system or scientific claim but rather a way of understanding psychedelic experience that pushes social science up to the edge of the abyss, the abyss that, as Nietsche said, also stares back at you. I am interested in playing with that edge but not going over it. I do that for very specific reasons, because I think that this approach speaks to a lot of people who are wary of, or otherwise not interested in, certain kinds of spiritual discourses. We can talk spirituality, we can talk alien beings, we can talk occult forces, we can even talk Jungian archetypes. But I think there are other ways of approaching these mysteries that some people are more amenable to. So I've been conscious of what I'm doing here in emphasizing the constructed character, the metabolic character, and the cultural human feedback loops that stage these encounters.

But those things are only *part* of the story, as we all know. In fact we can almost look at the entire visual dimension of the experience as a kind of interface, a kind of interface that we are co-creating in an encounter with something beyond, with something outside of these loops and stories. And that encounter is key for me. That's where all of the construction stories, all of the "Hey, our brains are making it up," and all of those self-reflexive critiques fall short. Because when I have an encounter with what Terence called the Other, existentially I don't need any ontology or any model of the world. I can have an encounter in a dream, I can have an encounter with a person on the street, I can have an encounter with an animal as I hike, and I can have an encounter with a marvelous appearance in a psychedelic trance. In my view, those encounters already contain within them demands that I must respond to—whether existentially, psychologically, imaginatively, or ethically—and just in terms of being an upright, appropriate person.

So in one sense I am encouraging an approach to these experiences with a certain skepticism, whether shamanic or psychonautical. It is good for visions to be distrusted, analyzed, put into a sociopolitical context, or to be appreciated and enjoyed, but it is also important for them to be set aside as sources of truth. At the same time what is also driving these thoughts are these encounters with enigmas that lurk beyond all that reflexivity; encounters that I cannot deny have already changed me and have already set me on splintering paths that contain further encounters and further initiations.

To boil it down here at the end, I'm not terribly interested in the content of visions. Now, I love the visions, but people overfetishize them. There's something else going on—maybe it's energetic, or interdimensional, or cosmic, or biophysical, or deconstructive. Are the elves a strange kind of animated interface that allows my brain to model my own neural processes? Maybe. But I still have to affirm the encounter, I can't avoid the encounter. And for me that possibility, that intuitive conviction, is what pulls all of this out of a merely reductive way of talking about visionary experience. But again this is just one model. I very much appreciate your attention, and I look forward to the questions.

Thank you.

DISCUSSION OF
How to Think about Weird Beings

WILL ROWLANDSON: Thank you. I've just had the most lovely experience of sitting for an hour and understanding profoundly and resonating with every word you've just said; it's been really fun . . .

ERIK DAVIS: I was particularly glad that you were here, because I knew that you would resonate with that.

ROWLANDSON: But there was just one little ripple on the fabric . . .

DAVIS: Sure.

ROWLANDSON: . . . and it's kind of stuck there and that was the metabolic envelope. In a way I only see that insofar as, for example, you might meet somebody for coffee because the entities are far more than a metabolic envelope, in the sense that some of the encounters I've had in a particular metabolic experience, such as the Hattifatteners in a Moomin book, are more than a metabolic experience. I also encountered elves and goblins and hobgoblins in the stories I was reading to my children; you see gargoyles on a church that are part of a dream, or a vision, or an experience that you had. So in that respect then, there's this constant interplay between different modes and different activities that you're engaged with and all these experiences you're having. Do you follow my question there?

DAVIS: I think I do, and I would say I'm in full agreement with you. You're interested in this notion of the metabolic arc of the experience and how that relates to the fact that the elements and the beings within this experience are clearly part of a larger, at least cultural, network that goes through time. For me these aren't separate issues. If we look at the network as already existing, that being the cultural network including our own experiences and images and even things that we don't necessarily know individually—and I do think this is where morphic resonance is certainly a very helpful idea, to explain certain things—that despite that network we should acknowledge and affirm the biophysical arc of the experience. No matter where these things are being drawn from, they are also unfolding and evolving through time. The network itself is in some ways sort of static, because that gargoyle has been there for five hundred years, so it's not going anywhere. Yet the way that it gets instantiated and signaled has this kind of developmental biophysical arc to it.

RICK STRASSMAN: It might be useful to consider a spectrum of metabolic cosmology to the entire package, because DMT is constantly being made and transported into the brain. It is probably mediating some narrow window of consensus reality. In addition, there's probably DMT being synthesized in the retina as well. So there may be more of a *spectrum* of the DMT worlds that we're encountering; with a narrow window of activity this is what we can see; then with higher levels it starts to move over to the other end of the spectrum, in more of a gradation rather than a categorical distinction.

DAVIS: Right, good.

JEREMY NARBY: Well, you worked with the dichotomy between science and enchantment, so science disenchants the world. Now we also know that questioning our dichotomies is often productive. Well, this one's pretty easy, because science has also enchanted the world, made it more interesting, and more mysterious. Many scientists have this kind of open-minded nondogmatic approach, and one can thank science for actually bringing many of the subjects we're discussing to the attention of the wider world. So what would be your comment on your own dichotomy?

DAVIS: Sure, sure. The boring answer is that it's simply expediency. In this situation saying "science" that way stands in for a lot of things that are really complicated, that take a long time to talk about, that combine materialism with modern industrial civilization, etcetera. But rather than say that, everyone knows this simple story: that "science comes along and completely disenchants the world." Because of course there's all these relations with religion as well as all the things that you're talking about. But I do like to set up that dichotomy, or something like that dichotomy, because to my mind it allows us to see the dialectics that are going in this space—the back and forth that fluctuates between these different ways of moving inside an experience, of taking it on and then standing away from it and critiquing it.

I mean that's already inside of spirituality, and it's already inside of science, that same dynamic. If you are a scientist and you have some hunch, where does it come from? Where do hypotheses come from— the inductive process, the deductive process, or the abductive process? So abduction, which is one way that people talk about the nature of forming hypotheses, is a mysterious thing; it's not easy to say exactly what's going on there, but certainly something like intuition is operating in the construction of a lot of hypotheses. So there you have it; already you have it inside science. And you have the other side of the equation inside religions; there's this process of questioning, of critique, of disenchantment. You have some remarkable experience in your past or whatever, and your pastor goes, "You might really want to work on that one a little bit more; here's a book to read, kid," or whatever it is. Spirituality also seems to include some kind of process of deconstructing your experience. So while I think it's a valid dichotomy, it's much more complicated than that.

STRASSMAN: I don't think it's even been a case of the processes themselves, but it could relate to the goals of science. In one of my favorite medieval biblical exegeses, Abraham Ibn Ezra likes to say that the goal of all of the sciences is God, so I think ultimately if you look at the goal of every science—biology, physics, astronomy, and mathematics even—it's been known as the source of the phenomenon.

DAVIS: Right. But the problem with science is not in the pursuit of knowledge, it's how the knowledge is plugged into all of these social, institutional, and economic forces. Most of the "science" that's done now is—whatever you want to call it—"techno-science." It's the production of something that might have value in a market; there's actually relatively little science where people are pursuing knowledge. You get that old sort of science still in astrophysics, you get it in some dwindling parts of botany, and with observers who are still out there looking at things . . .

DENNIS McKENNA: But that's why contemporary science is a caricature of science.

DAVIS: Right, yes, and in that sense there should be a better word; maybe that was not the right word to describe the dichotomy in that sense, because I'm certainly not interested in doing the typical bemoaning of science.

McKENNA: True science should be about the search for truth, a way to uncover true knowledge about the world. I think one of the main sort of spiritual or contemporary illnesses of science is that we've lost sight of that. Very few scientists ever take a course in philosophy of science. Very few scientists ever think about this. They're very good at their machines, and they can read charts and this sort of thing; they're not truth seekers, they're skilled technicians. But what's the purpose of science? The purpose of science is to have graduate students go to conferences, publish papers, get more grants, and do all this; the ultimate goal of science is completely obscured. To be a successful scientist, at least in the context of biomedicine in the United States, if somebody looked at you and said, "Why do you pursue this investigation?" and you said, "Well, it's to discover truth, it's to discover something about the way the world works," they'd look at you like you were nuts. Rick more than anyone else can say this. I mean it's not like he's been welcomed into the deepest halls of academe; he's been totally marginalized, because he has had the courage to ask questions that are not comfortable. And so that's a bit of a rant I did want to say.

I actually had a question, a remark on something that you said earlier, which I thought was very interesting. This notion of the spirit molecule, to bring these two words together is kind of an oxymoron: "Well, it's a molecule; how can it be spiritual?" But I think in light of what we've been talking about at this conference that's actually a completely reasonable thing. It is a spiritual molecule, a spirit molecule; it has a spirit quality because everything does. Everything's intelligent, and everything has a spiritual aspect, from electrons on up. So that's interesting. Then, on one hand you have the religious factions, or the sort of anti-religious factions but the pro-spirituality anti-religious factions, who can say, "Well, you know these religions boil down to psychedelics, so it's just a molecule, it's just drugs, man, it's just pharmacology, right?" You have that perspective, which doesn't acknowledge in fact that there's more going on because it does have a spiritual aspect; and then on the other hand you have biomedicine, and the psychedelics—particularly DMT—which have the potential to reintroduce spirit into medicine. Psychedelics therapeutically are basically used to treat spiritual illnesses on a cultural and individual level, so they are medicines for the soul and for the spirit, and biomedicine is absolutely terrified of them. Because in order to use those in biomedicine, biomedicine has to acknowledge that there is a spiritual aspect to medicine and healing, and the whole mechanistic model of healing goes out the window. In fact, they have to accept enchantment again, because they've spent four or five hundred years trying to exorcise that out of science. It creates a conundrum for both sides, which is right where we want to be.

DAVIS: Yes, the one dimension of that, which I wanted to talk about . . .

STRASSMAN: Well, the concept of intermediaries, which I'll talk about in my presentation, is a really useful one; intermediaries mediate between the spiritual and the physical, the incorporeal and the corporeal, so DMT could be looked at as an intermediary. The angels are considered as intermediaries between a physical world and a nonphysical God, and I think the notion of a spectrum is also useful in this context, in thinking of the spirit molecule. After I coined the phrase, a friend was reminded of a phrase in Genesis about mystics ascending from the earth before man was around to wander it. There's a cabalistic concept of the mist, which is kind of the gas in the blood, and he thought that DMT may have been, or might be, the mist. The way he phrased it was as the most spiritual of material and the most material of the spiritual.

DAVIS: Another dynamic that I didn't mention that I think is a real key to understanding Western psychedelic culture is the notion of the sacred and the profane together being a paradoxical driver of the spiritual path. Eliade made the sacred and the profane one of the key elements in his understanding of comparative religion—that there's the sacred and profane in any culture. It might have different qualities to it, but there's always this kind of distinction.

But Eliade was also very keen to emphasize that pretty much anything that you can imagine in the world, any part of the world, has at some point or another been identified by some culture or another as being sacred. In other words, stuff that most groups think of as profane is considered sacred by someone. So there's a weird tension between the sacred and the profane. They're not completely separated. And in fact they're kind of looped within each other. And I think a very key way of understanding psychedelic culture in the West is that it's loopy in precisely that way. It is playing with both sides.

Watching Graham St. John's presentation, we didn't go as far with it as I wanted to, which would be to go into the pop culture, the pop horror, and the Lovecraft, as well as the gaudiness that's in some of the psychedelic culture that he's looking at. If you think of some aspects of psytrance culture, or any number of things we can think of from the sixties, clearly we're not in anybody's conventional notion of the sacred. In fact sometimes it's explicitly driving against that into hedonism, into weirdness, into just being crazy, into a kind of antiauthoritarian move away from any traditional notion of the sacred. What do we do with all that stuff? Because threaded within that weirdness, that darkness—not even in dynamic opposition to it—is something of the sacred. And that tension, at least, seems to be very key because in a sense the sacred *is* the dynamic tension between the sacred and the profane.

GRAHAM ST. JOHN: I just wanted say that yours was a fabulous presentation. You evoked for me the significance in the psychedelic experience, of how compelling the psychedelic experience is. We're compelled to articulate the experience, we're compelled to write about it, we're compelled to produce trip reports and create art. Those are sacred processes, things like confession or, in the age of the internet, the confessions of

SWIM—Someone Who Isn't Me. We have these rhetorical moments that we can hang our confessions on. And so we have the spirit molecule, and we have those punkish elves, and we have the iconography that's provided by Alex Grey and so on. Richard Doyle—I don't know if you've read *Darwin's Pharmacy*—has some fabulous things to say about rhetoric and rhetorical modes in the psychedelic age.

DAVIS: Absolutely. Right. This makes me think of what happens when you look at the seventeenth and early eighteenth centuries, when this science stuff is getting going, when chemistry is trying to define itself against the alchemical tradition out of which it emerged. Individuals are very invested in making this division. One of the things they do to make this distinction is change their rhetoric. You begin to get the dry style—the telegraphed, nonpoetic way of describing an experiment or an event—which we all still use; that's part of the whole point. It happens in language; so in some ways that separation of science from the rest of human culture—which isn't ultimately a separation but changes everything nonetheless—occurs rhetorically. The poetic sensibility, which carries with it metaphor, resonance, allusion across time, different dimensions of language, and experience, gets whittled down to something that can be concretized and clarified. This is a major shift in scientific language. So I think our language around psychedelics is highly important and is a really important ethical dimension to keep in mind.

STRASSMAN: I was wondering how you understood Terence's statement about belief.

DAVIS: Well, as for Terence, that's a very good question. One of the things I'm interested in is that point where people approach what we would call religion or religious experience, but they also resist it in various ways or keep it at bay. One way to do that is to maintain a kind of naturalist perspective. And I think Terence was highly influenced by his love of Wallace, by his love of botany, and of natural history—I feel weird talking with Dennis here, but I'm just going to stay with Terence because it makes it easier . . .

McKenna: There's not a lot of difference.

Davis: I know, I mean, it's just weird anyway. Terence was very motivated by that model of the naturalist explorer, so he approached the DMT realm or the psychedelic realm as another *place*. It's like an unexplored continent, so we put on our pith helmets of awareness, we observe, and we pay attention to detail. These are all characteristics that I think grew out of his own naturalist temperament, being a rock hound and such when he was a young man and really glomming on to the model of the naturalist as the proper approach to these experiences as opposed to the spiritual approach.

I mean, Terence started doing this stuff at a time when everyone was turning to yoga and mysticism and Vedanta. And he's like "no." He's more interested in magic and alchemy than any of that stuff, and that's probably because magic is more like naturalism in a lot of ways, at least Western magic. And so that line about belief is his way of maintaining that perspective. He didn't want to get swallowed up in a particular belief system, even though of course in some ways he did. The Timewave was a belief that was incredibly important to him. We can't understand anything that he did without recognizing his need to hold on to, to reproduce, to keep working on, and reflecting on something that most people—including myself—see as a kind of cognitive fabulation, as something that doesn't hold real water for all sorts of reasons. That's okay, it doesn't bother me. It doesn't reduce my sense of Terence's brilliance or importance. There is a paradox there. Yet I still think his statement is true in a way, or it points to something significant about the way in which we balance a desire for enchantment and understanding and connection and encounter with a kind of sustained and skeptical disenchantment, which in a way is a kind of naturalist magic.

McKenna: Maybe a sign of a great mind is that you can hold contradictions in hand and be comfortable with that. What you're alluding to is the culture of Terence that I discussed in my talk yesterday with all of this amazing description of the phenomenology of experience; the last sentence was, "Yet we must investigate it in the usual way." Whatever that is. So that's the pith-helmet explorer doing that. There's a couple of things I'd like to say; for one, you know Terence had this belief system about the Timewave. I mean he was very invested in that, although I think maybe later in life he himself had serious doubts that people understood it perhaps as well as he did, which raised criticisms and his faith in that was shaken. But for many years he was involved in an illusion; I mean, I believe he believed it himself, he actually believed that the mushroom was an extraterrestrial entity. He would talk about the *Stropheria* and an age of the coming of the *Stropheria,* which is why when Jan Irving, for example, totally misinterprets it when Terence says, "Well, I worked for them underground for a long time and then they put me in PR." He was talking about the mushroom; he seriously believed that the mushrooms were an intelligent race or a channel to an intelligent race of beings, and he had a job with them—he was their ambassador. And he was, in a sense, but he was in a delusional space, though a benign enough delusional space. Maybe it wasn't a delusion. But then the other thing about the primacy of the encounter, the psychedelics, and the experience is that in some ways—I've said this and I think other people have too—psychedelics are an inoculum against faith. Faith is being asked to believe something where there's no evidence. You don't have to have faith to experience psychedelics. In fact, it's better if you don't. I imagine Rick will take issue with this, but it doesn't require faith; it simply requires receptivity and curiosity . . .

DAVIS: Practice and pay attention.

McKENNA: Have the encounter; make of it what you will.

ROWLANDSON: Dennis, that was a lovely little point that you raised there about living with a contradiction. There was a nineteenth-century

British ex-missionary in China, and he meets a guy and he asks, "Are you Confucianist or Taoist?" And the guy says, "Yep."

[Audience laughter.]

Erik, there was one issue that you raised that I think is really important. It's a point that I raised in the summer at the [Breaking Convention] conference . . .

Davis: Yes, I haven't seen that talk yet, but I've heard a lot about it.

Rowlandson: All right, the one issue I raise is the fact that you—we—all draw around this community of souls. We are here as a community of souls, our family, our friends, and our networks, and we draw to us people that we want to draw to us—as other people draw us to them—and we don't draw to us those types of beings that we would find really hostile and really unnegotiable, right? The same is true with all human beings; therefore, if we are setting ourselves up into a situation where we are taking seriously discussions, stories, and explanations of elves and the wee folk, we're talking about entities who do not want venerating. They don't want you to raise an altar and to organize the church of the heavenly elf, you know? They're going to trip you up and put your face in the custard tart. They're going to play with you and tie your shoelaces together. Every time you try to get too lofty and too theological, they're going to screw around with you. And consequently, it's by its own nature a contradiction in terms that there could ever be a solemn, somber communion of people celebrating in a somber place these funny little beings. Do you see? So I love the fact that in a way you have to keep your wits about you, you have to be alert, you can't abandon political thought, and you can't go in there saying, "Take me with you!" because they'll probably chuck you off a cliff. So you need to negotiate. You need to be alive, and aware, and present; I think that's what you were touching on when you were talking about Terence.

Davis: Yes, that's very well put, very well put.

NARBY: All this is true, but what is also true is that ayahuasca, for example, has lent itself to religion with great enthusiasm. Maybe you could comment on that?

DAVIS: I was just thinking the same thing and going, "Oh, that's a big question, maybe I'll not address it . . ." so you've forced my hand.

[Audience laughter.]

Of course there is religion in the whole picture, and I think Mestizo religions and practices are easier to talk about here because they're closer to the West in a lot of ways. They're already kind of deracinated in terms of indigeneity, and clearly there's this enormous panoply of relations, in that their practice is involved with healing. And then you get into this discussion about how we talk about religions where there is ungrounded faith, and yet they seem productive for lots of people. I'm not judgmental about things that work for people.

I'm more interested and more troubled by the way in which certain aspects of that religiosity come into the developed world. I'm wary of the way in which people sort of turn over their belief and think about these things simplistically, particularly with ayahuasca, where you have this whole neohippy world, and the shaman is the new guru. You can learn from shamans and gurus, but you should never worship them. And even that's okay, maybe. Even though I'm interested in describing this more skeptical trickster path, I'm very not critical of people's own ways through the mess, including profound religious belief and things that I have a great deal of respect for.

But I am interested in articulating a particular path where you may spend time in the mystery, you may go to the ceremony, you may discover these experiences without handing over your belief. I have my own gods, and I have had encounters that have changed me. I just don't talk about them because it's not really appropriate and not what I'm interested in talking about in a public discourse. But I have my own relations. It would be absurd for me to say, "Oh, these religions are deviations from this inherent encouragement from our psychedelic experiences to stay awake and keep on your toes." I'm really talking about a particular way of being in there, inside the trip, that I think is very important and central to my way of seeing things, but it isn't necessarily true for everyone, particularly if they're brought up in that culture. But I know Westerners who have gone deep into something like UDV*, and the problems and the beauty of that path represent the same kinds of things I see with other religions or occult belief systems that don't have a psychedelic basis.

McKenna: But every time you have a mysterium tremendum—a true spiritual mystery—somebody's going to try to co-opt it; isn't that essentially what's going on? Not just with ayahuasca, not just psychedelic religions, but anything?

Davis: Meditation too.

McKenna: I mean every organized religion wants to lay claim to it, since, you know, "we're the keepers, the guardians, and the only true institution that's honoring this real mystery." And that's why psychedelics are such a conundrum for religions, because that's their position. Then they turn around and do everything they can to suppress the actual encounter on an individual level with the true mystery. That's where the priests are; they're supposed to interpret things for you . . .

Davis: Yes, certainly, and it's always going to be there. So in a way I feel there's a middle path between these zones. There's an image at the end of *The Invisible Landscape* that talks about shamanism. I'm sure you have a different opinion about shamans than you did at that point, but it has always stayed with me. There's this image of the shaman as the tightrope walker through psychosis—it's a kind of materialist view, but it's a good one. There's something about the tightrope walker that accords with the way the world appears as I am talking about it right

---

*União do Vegetal, a spiritual organization dedicated to the sacrament of ayahuasca.

now. It's always in tension and in relation, and you kind of want to take a nap sometimes, but you've got to keep on the balance of the thing.

SHELDRAKE: Doesn't all religion involve encounters with entities? I'm religious myself; I pray on a daily basis, and if you pray, then you're actually inviting an encounter. In the Christian religion people pray to God, they pray to saints, and they pray to angels. In the Hindu religion you pray to all sorts of gods and goddesses. So in all religions there's this encounter as part of daily religious life, in the sense of forming a relationship or a connection.

DAVIS: I don't disagree with that at all. I'm not saying that this is the place where you get an encounter and in more ordinary religion it's just nonsense. But I do think that for many people in a religion, just as for many people who are psychedelic users, there isn't that degree of attention; rather there is a kind of just following along and not really dealing with the mystery before them. But there's always that vein of followers within religions that are very consciously—individually and collectively—cultivating these relationships that lead to real encounters that are transforming in the same ways that I was talking about. So I see these religions as sort of parallel in a way, but I'm also interested in this freethinking kind of spirituality. And that's more where I'm coming from.

SHELDRAKE: I think it's very interesting, but I think the context for a lot of people is a religious background where encounters with other beings are completely mainstream and standard, through prayer and so on.

MCKENNA: But is praying an encounter in itself? I mean, praying is sort of like sending a memo. If you get an answer back, you've got an encounter.

DAVIS: Well, let me offer an example. There's a wonderful book by an anthropologist named Tanya Luhrmann, and it's called *When God Talks Back*. In American evangelism, especially in the past thirty or forty years, there has been an emphasis on the personal relationship with Jesus and not in a general sense but literally, in terms of having that presence, that voice, that guiding voice within you. What Luhrmann talks about—a beautiful example of how you can simultaneously be true to a skeptical social-scientist view and still be extremely appreciative and supportive of people's religious experiences—is how people, as they move through their faith, have to *learn* how to listen for the "voice of God."

So you could say, "Well, they're just being acculturated," if you're being a skeptical social scientist. But from the inside it's also about a question of practice: how do people in the course of their spiritual lives develop the capacity to recognize, let's say, "voices in your head," as forms of relation with a being that has the force of encounter? Whatever the ontology is, it's something that's built through training. It's extremely real and existential.

MCKENNA: But if you didn't get an answer back at least occasionally it would be frustrating. You'd get tired; most people would give up eventually.

SHELDRAKE: I don't think most people experience prayer as just sending a request like an email and then hoping for an answer. I think they experience it as being—well, I can speak for myself—I experience it as being in the presence of God, and open to the divine, and like a conversation much more than sending an email.

MCKENNA: Does he answer back in a personal way?

SHELDRAKE: Yes, not through words, but through the sense of presence.

MCKENNA: Right.

STRASSMAN: Well, there are different kinds of prayer, but the request kind is a petition. You know, there are also prayers of thanksgiving, and there are prayers of grace; so prayers aren't only to request.

SHELDRAKE: No, quite. I agree. And there's contemplative prayer, which is very similar to meditation.

DAVID LUKE: I think probably just one last question.

ROBIN CARHART-HARRIS: I've been listening with an open mind since I've been here and more and more building up a feeling that I should say something in defense of what's sometimes referred to as a materialist approach. It's an unfortunate term, sort of sounds like materialist as in the acquisition of material goods. In terms of hearing you talking about the dry language that you will find in scientific literature, I want to frame that slightly differently. I want to say that what we aim to do as scientists is to be dispassionate, to really give ourselves the best chance to glean what is true. I also want to argue against the idea that scientists are only after getting the next publication or the next grant. I'm here with an open mind; I'm interested in these entity experiences that can be induced by DMT. I want to say my motivation is one of pragmatism as a scientist. I want to hear the phenomenology, I want to be systematic, I want to be pragmatic in my approach, and I want to test these ideas. I want to put them to the test and use that model as a way to glean truth. What worries me slightly about a desire for enchantment is that there's something wishful as well as basking or luxuriating, I suppose, in mystery and enchantment, which is fine. As I say, I come here with an open mind wanting to understand the phenomena but with a motivation to try to study it. I think if you just leave it in this enchanting space, then you might be motivated not to even study it. So I just wanted to put my cards on the table.

DAVIS: I'm very glad you represented that here. That's why I really try to emphasize how, both in terms of intellectual work and in terms of spiritual work, that disenchantment—analysis, critique, thinking hard, breaking things down, whatever you want to call that—has always been equal in my life to enchantment. One without the other is kind of lost in some sense. And the point about dry is not to say, "Oh, it's dry; science is missing the thing"; it's really just to say that part of the enormous productivity and all of the knowledge that came, once we got science rolling, had to do with a rhetorical decision and the way of organizing and reproducing language. So that dispassionate quality, which is deeply tied in with science, emerges fully from Christianity and is also deeply Christian. In many ways, you can't understand the origins of science without really understanding Christianity, including that dispassionate character.

Many of the pious ideals of science emerged from Christianity and then were transformed as they moved off and started operating on their own. So when I hear you talking I hear the ethics of science and the ethics of the pursuit of knowledge; I also still hear—not enchantment, that's not the right word—a more-than-indifferent interest in facts. I hear that kind of call, and the move toward dry language is part of the practice. It's the way that Theravada Buddhism is extraordinarily dry. You read these descriptions, and they are incredibly dry. Why? Because the language represents perhaps the most direct way to deconstruct the ego that exists in the world traditions. It *has* to be dry. It's not about enchantment; it's about breaking down the delusions of self. So I just want to say that I respect very much that language and that move and the dispassionate quality that you're talking about.

STRASSMAN: One can look for enchantment; I think one can study enchantment through rigorous methodology. I mean, my DMT study was phrased in the most dry, banal psychopharmacological terms possible, but ultimately it was my intent to bring enchantment into the discussion of the mind in psychiatry.

LUKE: With that, thank you, Rick, and thank you, Erik.

CHAPTER 6

Why May DMT Occasion Veridical Hallucinations and Informative Experiences?

EDE FRECSKA

I am very grateful for being here, but at the same time I feel disheartened because today I heard presentations about how difficult it is to make statements on psychedelics. I feel somewhat vulnerable because I will come up with strong statements about psychedelics. The challenge I am putting myself against is to interpret how come we can get sometimes reliable information from anomalous sources, in an anomalous way. Anomalous, because it doesn't fit into that kind of "gaining knowledge" process that is accepted in Western thinking. It's an anomalous source, because it is based on the use of psychedelics.

It is a shamanic practice in the Amazon Basin: the curandero, or native healer, puts the leaves of a plant into the hallucinogenic ayahuasca brew, and in this way he or she will get in touch with the spirit of the plant and can attain knowledge about its healing potential. In the anthropological records, one can read that a Siberian shaman may find lost objects or in Bushman settlements when the women and children—who were left behind while the men went on a hunt—knew in advance when the hunters would return and would make the necessary preparations for their welcome. These are phenomena one may call anomalous, since Western academic thinking cannot interpret such reports and chooses to ignore them.

Let us discuss another topic that was in the title of our symposium: plant sentience. Western science is at the very beginning of accepting that plants may have intelligence. It may take Western academia a long time to realize and acknowledge how much sentience plants may have. Moreover, more time and research is needed for the acceptance that we humans are capable of accessing plants' knowledge in a way similar to the curanderos: with the help of the ayahuasca brew or some other shamanic practice.

Therefore, I am proposing a second foundation of knowledge for the interpretation of anomalous phenomena. I am fully aware that dichotomizing is a problematic issue. Regardless, I think it's more troublesome if Western thinking doesn't notice that we Westerners are dichotomizing, and we are totally tied to one side of a duality. When I presented this kind of concept to a Kabbalist rabbi or Sufi monk I got the response: "We know that knowledge has two foundations," and they added, "However, eventually knowledge is One."

Contemporary Western thinking is based on one side of a duality. Two ways of knowledge were proposed by Parmenides of Elea, a Greek pre-Socratic thinker who is known as the Father of Logic and the "first mover" of Western rational thinking. However, the West has followed only one side of his teaching.

Today I will offer a similar dichotomy, but I have no clue how to glue the two sides together to be One. Therefore, I will just present to you how dualism appears in the way of seeking truth. At the same time, I would like to convince you about the complementarity between the two ways of knowledge.

In essence, what I am proposing here is that we are able to get a representation of the outside environment in two different ways. These two ways of representation follow the dual nature of the physical universe: locality and nonlocality. Locality means energy exchange when the information is coming from space-time constraints. In these cases, particles hit the sensory organs and the information goes through cognitive processing. In a juxtaposition, I propose another way of making representation of the outside world based on nonlocality. On this path I am against British empiricism by stating that information may reach the brain without going through the senses. In order to interpret mystic teachings and shamanic lore, one must suppose that information processing may bypass the senses. However, as I will show, it doesn't bypass the body. Based on the model presented, the body serves as some sort of *quantum array antenna* by getting nonlocal information via quantum correlations from the environment.

This interpretation is not about left- and right-brain dichotomy. Basically, it's not about the dominance of the left over the right hemisphere. Actually, it is about an up and down dichotomy between neuro-axonal and subcellular levels while addressing information processing in the brain and in the body. I propose here a neuro-ontological interpretation of spiritual experience. I go further than many scholars who accept spiritual ideas but usually stop at the epistemological level. Usually, they try to avoid discussing the ontological background of these experiences—which is what I am going to do.

During an inner journey the shaman goes somewhere, and it's striking that he brings back information, which he then uses to improve the well-being of the community. From a systems theory perspective, the shaman is a reintegrator: he improves the integration of the system. It is not possible to reorganize a dysfunctional system from the inside. One can only do it by getting restructuring information from the outside. So what is the source of the shaman's information? It must be nonlocal according to my answer.

Very probably, neurons are not the only building blocks of information processing, and consciousness is not emerging from neuroaxonal activity. Why not? We know that there is the observer paradox in quantum physics: the observer's decision influences the outcome of the physical experiment. Then how is it that an electrochemical organ like the brain can influence quantum processes? The assumption that every human experience results from the activity of one network, the neuro-axonal, may turn out to be a fallacy of neuroscience. Francis Crick was bold enough to say, "You are nothing but a pack of neurons." It is a rudely radical reductionism, not because it's materialistic, as psychoanalysis can be radical, saying, "You are nothing but a bunch of neurotic complexes," but that is reductionism too.

Theories based on classical physics are insufficient to explain who we are. That is another fallacy of current neuroscience. It's interesting that more than fifty years ago, within two years after discovering cosmic background radiation, physicists and astronomers accepted quantum concepts in explanation of the macrocosmos. As far as the microcosmos is concerned, we are not there yet, despite the important initial steps of Stuart Hameroff and some others who have introduced quantum mechanics into neuroscience. In addition, you can read a lot in New Age literature about "the quantum mind"—well, the quantum sells very well. My contribution to this stream is discussing how quantum effects may reach the brain; what is the interface between the quantum world and the mind?

How do I approach this challenge? I cannot follow the typical scientific way—experimental and so on, not even using others' theoretical ideas incorporated into mine—because it's such an uncharted territory. Instead I am using what I would call the "attorney's approach," though I've never been an attorney, so perhaps attorneys wouldn't like what I'm saying. I suppose that a good attorney doesn't have to know necessarily what the case is really; in order to win, it is enough for her to reveal the inconsistencies of the other party's statements.

Therefore, I'm trying to point out what inconsistencies we have in the Western approach. I like that epistemological consideration according to which everything is about narration: we are making stories.

Even in science, we are generating narrations; theories are narrations, or stories, that follow certain rules, which I call the "Rules of four C." Within two narrations or two theories, one is better: the one that is more Comprehensive, Congruent, Compact, or better Connected to other fields of knowledge. I like the fourth one—this is what I'm using here—because I try to connect Western thinking to mystical thinking. For example, from a pragmatic point of view, the Ptolemaic and Copernican worldview were equal, but the Copernican worldview better fulfilled the fourth rule: it was better connected to other fields of knowledge.

My goal is to come up with a good story by following the Rules of four C. Against the fallacy of neuroscience, my counterproposal sounds like this: we are more than one network. Usually I hate the holographic principle because New Age literature is abusing it, but regardless, I have to refer to it. Matti Pitkänen—the Finnish physicist—said, "The universe emulates itself on every level." Statements like this can illustrate what I am trying to do by translating into Western language what is said by mystical teaching or indigenous people. This statement, "the universe emulates itself on every level," is a contemporary version of the hermeneutic wisdom "as above, so below." My basic tenet is: at the bottom or the top—it doesn't matter where we enter nonlocal realms—there is a nonbiological web embedding our existence and consciousness nonlocally in the universe.

Discussing the principle of nonlocality may take a lot of time. Please look into it elsewhere, since this is an emerging and complicated concept. I can only address it here briefly. Over the last twenty years the principle of nonlocality has grown up as the second pillar of quantum mechanics. The other pillar is Heisenberg's Uncertainty Principle. Nonlocality means that elementary particles, which were part of the same quantum system, remain connected even after apparent separation. So their states remain in correlation with each other. For example, after gamma decay, an electron goes one way and a positron goes the other way. It is still one quantum system. So if you change the spin of one, according to [Max] Planck, the spin of the other must change instantaneously regardless of how far apart they are. Albert Einstein said that this is spooky action at a distance, and he tried to refute it. In the early '80s, Alain Aspect's team, followed by John Archibald Wheeler's, was able to show that this is really the case: entangled elementary particles maintain their connection with each other after separation.

For parapsychologists, nonlocality comes to the rescue as an explanation of psi phenomenon. However, the second pillar of quantum mechanics, the uncertainty principle, makes their research and replication difficult: sometimes this kind of interaction comes up with fuzzy results. Therefore, if I try to use quantum correlations to explain some anomalous phenomena, I have to admit that at times their spooky effect can be pretty obscure and unreliable.

Considering the levels of organization relevant to consciousness from society and culture down to the Planck scale, I would like to point out that there is an arbitrary line in the middle, between the synaptic and the cytoskeletal level [see figure 1]. Above that line, there is a bottom-up and top-down interaction at work between the levels. For example, culture can shape how our neuroaxonal network will be nourished, and the makeup of our neuroaxonal network has some impact on what kind of society and community we build. So there are top-down and bottom-up interactions at work in the upper field. Also above the dotted line, from neurons up to culture, we have good theories about how every level gives something to human experience. Below the line, from the cytoskeleton down to the Planck scale—what the current mainstream view supposes—there are just servient, subdominant levels. They just make the other layers above the line functional, and there is not too much top-down or bottom-up interaction between them, and what is more, they give nothing specific to our consciousness.

Diverging from neuroscientific views that tie consciousness to neuroaxonal activity, I suppose that these lower levels also add something to human consciousness, and this is nonlocality. They are able to

higher?
  culture/society
    organism/brain/personality
      subpersonalities/unconscious complexes
        "sub-brains" (hemispheres, MacLean's triune brain)
        cortico-thalamic feedback loops
        brain modules/neural networks
        neurons/axons
          synapses/neural membranes
----
        microtubular network
        microfilamental lattice
        citosol
          protein complexes
            hydrophobic packets
              van der Waals (London) forces
                electron superpositions/photon polarizations
                space-time geometry (Akashic field?)

Figure 1. Organizational levels that play a role in human experiences.

bring in nonlocal influences, or interactions. But on what level can they do that exactly?

If one considers the neuroaxonal level, it's pretty "macro" for quantum events. Stuart Hameroff supposed that the microtubular system could serve as a medium for quantum computation, but he didn't discuss nonlocality in his theory. Microtubuli create a vast system, much vaster than the neuroaxonal: there are ten million times more building blocks in the microtubular system. Nevertheless, it's not minuscule enough for nonlocal interactions. There is another system that is finer than the microtubular, and that is the microfilamental network, or the intracellular lipoprotein membrane system. This system is one huge continuous membrane—because the vast majority of the body's cells are connected with each other through gap junctions—and this membrane is microscopic enough to maintain quantum correlations with the environment. Somewhere at this level I propose a quantum array antenna network, which receives some nonlocal effect and can serve as a medium for a holographic representation of the environment.

I can hardly pinpoint what cellular structure provides that interface. Therefore, in the rest of my presentation I will refer to this as the subcellular system, and I'll refer to the other system as the neuroaxonal, which according to the relativistic view is the only network that makes us human.

Earlier I mentioned duality and complementarity in the physical universe, according to which there is a local and nonlocal dichotomy. Here I propose a duality and complementarity in knowledge by adding a second foundation of knowledge, based on nonlocality. With the help of the subcellular quantum array antenna, our body is in contact with the whole Universe. I say body because probably it's not only our brain. Our body may contain the whole cosmos like a hologram, which would support the truths of "the Kingdom of Heaven is within you," and "look into yourself; you are Buddha," or "as without, so within."

We can get knowledge by turning outside; this is the local way of learning, but the nonlocal way of learning is the opposite; you are turning inside. In the Nested Network model of human experience [see figure 2], the brain's sensory inputs are local effects and involve energy exchange. In addition to this sensory input, there is a hologram within the body, depending on nonlocal quantum correlation with the outside world.

I try to avoid the term "entanglement," because entanglement is a specific form of quantum correlation. Current theories that start to speak about "quantum discord" can also be the basis of quantum information.

Stuart Hameroff and Roger Penrose's theory implies that if the structure of a protein molecule changes due to energy exchange with other molecules, then there must be a corresponding change in mass according to Einstein's special theory of relativity. If there is a mass change, then there must be a wrinkle in space-time, according to Einstein's general theory of relativity. One may say this is an infinitesimally little change, but quantum mechanics tells us how small changes can exert very profound effects. The main point here: life is about

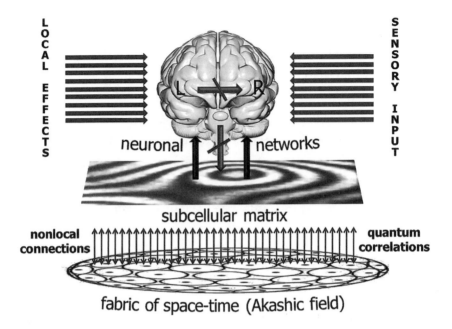

Figure 2. Nested networks with two inputs.

continuous energy exchange; due to energy exchange there is change in mass, and that mass change makes an imprint in a nonbiological network outside of us. This way we are out of the realm of biological systems, and what is happening inside us makes an imprint within the physical realm, especially in the fabric of space-time. Penrose calls this web, down at the Plank scale, a "spinor network." Ervin Laszlo named it differently: the "Akashic holofield." Regardless, naming doesn't change the concept.

According to the Nested Network model, the neuroaxonal brain is coping machinery for the purpose of quickly responding to environmental challenges—that's why it had to rely on the certain, local effects. The model assumes a second network serving another representation of the outside world and providing different knowledge, but usually in the ordinary state of consciousness it is the brain, the coping machinery, that dominates. In some altered states of consciousness—for example, the shamanic state of consciousness—and after the use of certain techniques, this dominance is eliminated.

One way is to frustrate the coping machinery by overloading it with stressful stimuli. The best example is the Lakota Sioux Sun Dance where the participants are exposed to several kinds of physical and mental stress. After hours and days of the arduous ceremony, the coping machinery gives up. It is similar to the process when the left hemisphere, unable to handle a visual-spatial task, gives it up and decreases its dominance over the right brain—which has a more intimate relationship with the body than the left—but in this case the dominance is not within one network, neuroaxonal, but rather is between network, neuroaxonal versus subcellular.

Another way is the use of Zen koans, which mentally frustrate this coping machinery until it gives up and steps aside. There is something similar, I suppose, about psychedelics. Dimethyltryptamine [DMT] and other psychedelics may shift information processing from the neuroaxonal toward the subcellular level. The most difficult technique is to get rid of the dominance of the brain by yoga meditation.

What else can be understood with the help of the Nested Network model? Out-of-body experience [OBE] can be conceptualized in terms of the Nested Network, as awareness is scanning inside the holographic matrix, within the representation of the environment that is in the body. And sometimes an OBE can get relevant information. We have anecdotal reports of people who while in OBEs saw objects that they were not supposed to see.

Another interpretation may come from this model: for example, how come shamans and other healers can see auras? What are auras? From my point of view, auras are some sort of synaesthesia. In synaesthesia, two sensory modalities are combined. For example, someone sees a brown sound. If a sensory modality—visual in this case—is blended with nonlocal information in a synaesthesia-like relationship, then that can give emergence to auras, or spirits, or perhaps even DMT entities.

In the table that follows, the left side is the perceptual-cognitive way of knowledge—this is what we usually consider as a way of knowledge—and the right side is what I call the direct-intuitive mode. Direct because it passes the senses, and intuitive because intuition is the closest to what this knowledge channel is about. You can notice that one way of knowledge is essentially learning by observation from the outside; this is the objective, scientific way of learning. On the right side, there is learning by observation from the inside. As I addressed earlier, this channel opens when you are not looking and going outside for information; instead you go deep inside yourself and may get information not only about self, but also about what is in the outside world.

DUALITY AND COMPLEMENTARITY IN KNOWLEDGE

Perceptual-Cognitive (rational)	Direct-Intuitive (visionary)
Hylotropic mode	Holotropic mode
Learning by observation from the outside (objective)	Learning by observation from the inside (subjective)
Neuroaxonal network is the medium (in the brain)	Subcellular matrix is the medium (in the body)
Electrochemical (based on local effects)	Quantumphysical (based on nonlocal connections)
Performs modeling, splits to subject-object	Direct experience, no subject-object split
Linguistic (not necessarily verbal), transferable	Ineffable, nontransferable (but can be directly shared)
Precise, it has little problems with replicability	Nebulous, it has big problems with replicability
Peaks in Western scientific thinking	The source of contemplative (and shamanic) traditions

In essence, you go deep down enough and in this way you will be out; that's why we gave the title to our book with Rick Strassman, *Inner Paths to Outer Space.* If you go inside you can get outside, and you may get some veridical information. The perceptual-cognitive mode is also based on the electrochemical effect, whereas the direct-intuitive mode, as I suppose, is quantum physical, nonlocal. The first one performs modeling and splits awareness into subjects and objects, and the second one provides direct experience—there is no subject-object split, and it is ineffable. The first one is linguistic. Even the nonverbal, right hemisphere is linguistic—we know about artistic language, we've heard about musical language—but this direct-intuitive mode is free of any language.

Two mystics can probably understand each other much better than two climatologists, because language and model are bypassed. But they also have egos, so sometimes it doesn't work too well.

The direct-intuitive mode is ineffable and nontransferable. Basically, what we do in schools is transferring knowledge, but this kind of intuitive knowledge cannot be transferred. That's why it has dropped out of Western education. On the other hand, while it is ineffable, you can point at it. When Michael Harner discussed his experience with a Conibo shaman, the shaman knew what he was talking about. You cannot pass it on or transfer it to others, but you can agree that you probably had a similar experience.

There is a peculiar feature of this second way of knowledge: you can have shared visions, you can have shared consciousness, and you can have the same vision. Shared consciousness and shared inner experiences are testable. However, this intuitive way is so nebulous that it has big problems with replicability, and that's why Big Science ignores it. Many scientists realize measuring things is not the *sine qua non* of science, but scientists are definitely tied to replicability. I would quote George Carlin: "Drop your need, buddy!"

I have heard from Jeremy Narby and Christian Ratsch that we can hardly understand pre-Columbian South American civilizations just starting out from Western thinking. Well, understanding the "learning by observation from the inside" may get us closer.

Duality and complementarity as a double principle can be found elsewhere. Visual perception has two channels, two modes. One is the "what or who" channel; it follows a totally different neural pathway than the other one, the "where and how." The "what" channel is the focal, the sharp; the "where and how" channel is the peripheral. Both are very important for survival. People with tunnel vision lack the peripheral retinal input. It is very difficult to live in tunnel vision. From my perspective, if Western science is entirely tied to the perceptual-cognitive way of knowledge, that can result in a sort of tunnel vision. Intuitive knowledge can provide very important ideas that we can follow through scientifically. In the *Rig Veda,* one may find very interesting ideas about the world, some similar to the concepts of quantum physics. Using the metaphor above, the *Rig Veda* represents the peripheral vision. However, one cannot build a transistor or microchip based only on the teaching of the Vedas; for that goal, one needs the focal approach of the scientific method. My point is: Western civilization is in strong need of using both ways of knowledge in a complementary manner.

What, or who, are the DMT entities? According to this model, some DMT entities and spirits are informative components of the nonlocal domain that are brought into the perceptual-cognitive processing in a culturally specific manner. They are quasi-autonomous structures; "quasi-" because they have some autonomy but are basically belief systems; our expectations have a morphing-plastering effect on them. And not only ours—for people from the past and future who had or will get into contact with them, their expectation shapes them because they are in a nonlocal realm; so not only *current* cultural expectations may be influential. Entities emerging from the nonlocal domains may have veridical potencies, or not; as you know, they are tricksters, so most of these encounters are uninformative. For many they can be totally misleading, and getting reliable information via divination needs a shaman or an initiated person.

The visions have a role in shaping our culture because healing, art, religion, civilization, philosophy, logic, and mathematics all had some visionary experience at their roots. For millennia shamanic healing was performed in visionary shamanic states of consciousness. As we know from David Lewis-Williams, shamanic trance was the origin of Paleolithic art. Regarding religion, prophetic visions were first, scriptures came next. Civilization was my third chapter in Rick Strassman's book. I wrote there that the Anunnakis were probably imaginary-visioned beings who provided the Sumerians with the knowledge that *we* got from Sumerians: written language, school systems, legal systems, metallurgy, shipbuilding, and so forth. The Sumerians learned all of it from the Anunnakis—as they stated themselves. I would like to point out another inconsistency of Western thinking: we admire Sumerians, what we got from them, but when we get to the point of how they explain the source of this knowledge, we don't care.

Regarding logic, Parmenides of Elea had a shamanic journey—probably underworld, according to Peter Kingsley—when he met with the goddess who provided him the necessity of logical argumentation, which was the basis of Aristotelian logic. And don't forget the father of mathematics, Pythagoras, who was called a shaman, because *iatromantis* in Greek has a similar meaning, like shaman, a miracle healer. Aristotle wrote somewhere that, according to his mates, they saw him at the same time at different places, and he was supposed to talk to animals. He got his knowledge by divination. This is not what the father of mathematics is supposed to do—this is a shaman's task. René Descartes, the founder of European rational philosophy, had three dreams as motivators.

In conclusion, we have duality and complementarity in culture because intuitive visions and insights create culture, and language transfers it. They are equally important. However, I have seen more doctoral dissertations about language than about visions, so this is out of balance.

At last, these are some thoughts on artificial intelligence [AI], plants, and information processing. In the AI department, what they try to model is only perceptual-cognitive thinking. I don't assume that AI researchers are studying the direct-intuitive way—while they use it in person—or are working on how to incorporate this second channel into AI. I have heard that Alan Turing had among his principles the idea that the perfect AI should have telepathic experiences, but of course, it was wiped out later on. You can hear from leading scientists: "The brain can be downloaded into a chip." Not mine. I suppose that one has to model the whole universe back to the Big Bang in order to perform such endeavours, since mankind and animals use the nonlocal channel as well.

Are there creatures that can only use the direct-intuitive? Those are the plants, I assume. They don't have this neuroaxonal network, so they will not tell you. Don't expect a plant to talk to you in words, but what if we were able to tune in to this direct-intuitive mode of information collecting, using our nonlocal way, to get in contact with them?

The *Populus tremuloides* has a huge root system, as much as six million kilograms, which you can call one organism. Marine plants like *Posidonia oceanica* can have an extension of several miles and estimated age of about one hundred thousand years. A mushroom specimen called *Armillaria ostoyae* found in the state of Washington has a couple of square miles of mycelia network. It is possible that plants have enormous information processing ability, but not the one we usually describe, not the neuroaxonal and electronic, but another type, perhaps nonlocal. There must be huge, vast information-processing power in plant knowledge that one can be informed about in an ayahuasca, DMT, or psilocybin experience, and this is what South American shamans use as a source of information.

Duality and complementarity in living nature is amazing. Consider modularity and singularity. Plants are modular; after losing 99 percent of its body, a plant can regrow, but at the same time they are singular, because they have tight junctions, so a plant can be considered and function like a single cell. We animals are somewhere in between. We follow the rule of "organicity." Our life is based on organs and individuality, but plants are "dividuals." Plants perform extremely well on these two ends, modularity and singularity, and they are the perfect embodied agents.

The best concluding remarks are these citations from revered authors:

The Universe is emulating itself in all length and time scales and it is quite possible that quantum computations are carried out in all relevant biological length scales.

MATTI PITKÄNEN,
FROM *TOPOLOGICAL GEOMETRODYNAMICS*

The mycelium is an exposed sentient membrane, aware and responsive to changes in its environment. . . . Interlacing mycelial membranes form, I believe, a complex neuron-like web that acts as a fungal collective consciousness.

PAUL STAMETS, FROM *MYCELIUM RUNNING:
HOW MUSHROOMS CAN HELP SAVE THE WORLD*

The mushroom consciousness is the consciousness of the Other in internal link hyperspace, which means in dream and in the psilocybin trance, at the quantum foundation of being, in the human future, and after death.

TERENCE MCKENNA, FROM *FOOD OF THE GODS:
THE SEARCH FOR THE ORIGINAL TREE OF KNOWLEDGE—
A RADICAL HISTORY OF PLANTS, DRUGS,
AND HUMAN EVOLUTION*

These thoughts help to understand why people of the Amazon Basin turn to plant teachers like ayahuasca, and why their answer to the Jesuit question, "How do you know what you know?" is, "From the plants."

DISCUSSION OF
Why May DMT Occasion Veridical Hallucinations and Informative Experiences?

BERNARD CARR: Well, I'd like to make a couple of comments. First of all, I was very glad that you mentioned the link with physics. I think I'm probably one of the only physicists here, so I was obviously very pleased to relate to that, but also I was very pleased with the way in which you expanded the discussion from just looking at DMT to a whole variety of other sorts of anomalous psychic-type experiences.

I'm interested in psychical research, and it's clear that it's a common feature of many psychic experiences that one is encountering a different level of reality, a different type of intelligence, one that's nonmaterial. I do think if you're trying to have a theory of these psychedelic-type experiences, then you have to see it in the context of a broader range of phenomena. Rupert [Sheldrake] mentioned encounters in prayer—that's another example. I think that's very important.

I would like to respond a bit to your comments about the role of quantum theory being the basis of such a theory. It is clear that quantum theory is the one part of physics where consciousness somehow creeps in, so I think it's undoubtedly true that whatever our final theory is, quantum theory—and concepts of entanglement and nonlocality that you referred to—will play a crucial role. But I would like to caution against a view in which that's the be-all and end-all, the final explanation, because no one understands quantum theory anyhow, and merely saying it can be explained by quantum theory is just replacing one mystery with another mystery.

What you really need is a more fundamental theory that explains consciousness and mentality as well as quantum theory. Now the question is: What is the nature of that theory? I'd just like to sort of push my own approach, although it isn't a mainstream approach from physicists. It seems to me that what is interesting and what is in common with all these experiences, including the psychedelic- and DMT-type experiences, is that they involve some form of space. And it's also true that many psychic phenomena, out-of-body experiences, dreams, and apparitions—almost the entire gamut of psychic phenomena—do involve some form of space.

It seems to me that if you want to link that to some physical theory, then it's the existence of that space that is really crucial. As some people may know, I've been pushing my own view for quite a while, which basically says that physics teaches us that space is more than just the three dimensions of space and the one dimension of time; there are these extra dimensions that are now almost taken for granted by physicists, and it's always seemed to me that those higher dimensions can play a crucial role in accommodating these different forms of reality.

The main problem with the materialistic reductionist view of physics is that it says there is only one form of reality; it's this reality of three dimensions of space and the one dimension of time. That's what you've got to get away from—the notion that there is only one level of reality. If you accept that the only level of reality is this material world, then you also accept that all these other levels of reality that you encounter in out-of-body experiences, near-death experiences, and psychedelic trips are all illusions. But once you allow the possibility that the final picture of reality involves these extra dimensions, then you have the possibility of many levels of realities, like a hierarchy of levels of realities, which is in principle able to accommodate all of these sorts of phenomena. That's why I listen with particular interest when people talk about types of space and intelligences within those spaces, which are encountered within these drug experiences. Seems to me they give a vital clue as to what the nature of that space is.

EDE FRECSKA: Let me give you this example. I outlined two ways of information processing. For comparison, let's say they correspond to two operating systems. Every operating system has its own environment. One operating system is the perceptual-cognitive, and its environment is this perceptual reality, where the principle of action-reaction applies. The reality of the other, or the intuitive, is a different reality. Different kinds of reality crop up according to the two different approaches. Multidimensionality can be tricky. Jim DeKorne had a thought experiment: imagine a two-dimensional being who is yelled at from a three-dimensional space. Where will this two-dimensional creature hear the voice? According to DeKorne, it will arise as hallucination from the inside.

CARR: You see, when you talk about this inner and outer way of gaining information about the universe, which I agree with, normally people are only applying that to the physical world, in the sense that you're getting information about the physical world either externally through telescopes and particle accelerators or internally through some form of clairvoyance or drug experience. But the point is, that's the *mode* of perceiving reality, but that's different and not quite the same as the nature of reality itself. And the point is, your inner mode of perception is, I would say, also accessing a level of reality that is not accessed by the normal external approach. That's my view.

DAVID LUKE: I loved how you applied this approach to the basis of culture, and how all these different things like healing and the arts come through this intuitive process. It's probably good to remind ourselves that the basis of modern Western medicine was actually founded on the ancient dream temple tradition.

FRECSKA: The cult of Asclepios and their practice of dream incubation; that's fascinating, yes.

LUKE: Exactly, so that's certainly one good example of it.

FRECSKA: The snake was the healer. Yes.

LUKE: And that's where we get several medical words too, *clinic* and *therapy,* and so on.

FRECSKA: *Therapeuts* were the dream interpreters, and *clinié* was the altar, yes.

LUKE: Many things like that. I think that's all we've got time for; thank you very much, Ede.

DAY THREE

■ ■ ■ ■ ■

Exploring the Whole of Reality

On this day we'll hear from four speakers. First, Andrew Gallimore, neurobiologist, pharmacologist, and chemist, will discuss the nature of reality as we know it and the nature of the reality of the DMT world—including how these worlds evolved and whether or not they are mutually exclusive. Next, biologist Rupert Sheldrake will discuss the rediscovery of the world around us from the perspective of morphic resonance and collective memory, the idea that those who take psychedelics may be unconsciously influenced by those who have taken them in the past. Both talks attempt to expose how reality is created. Graham Hancock, spiritually minded author and public figure, will discuss commonalities between fairy, elf, and alien abductions, both ancient and modern, to show that the reality of these worlds is not so dissimilar, and in fact they overlap with DMT experiences. Our talks will conclude with a presentation from Rick Strassman, psychiatrist and psychopharmacologist, who will defend why the DMT world may be as real if not more real than everyday reality and will offer a theoneurological roadmap to further exploration.

The day was one of exploration, and we debated what experiments and what sojourns into unknown territory might be undertaken in the future to continue to advance our knowledge.

The Neurobiology of Conscious Interaction with Alternate Realities and Their Inhabitants

Andrew Gallimore

Although I kind of feel now like I'm among friends, most, or many of you, when I arrived probably wouldn't have known who the hell I was, and I'm acutely aware that I'm heading up quite a lineup today, so I should introduce myself. What I normally do is jump up and down rather impishly in front of my slide show; I was born in the city of Lincoln, and the symbol of Lincoln is the imp, and I have been called the Lincoln imp. Actually the first thing that Peter [Meyer] said to me when he met me on Monday was, "Has anybody ever told you that you look like an elf?" Thanks for that. What I will try to do is slow it down and do this from a seated position, but if I jump up at some point and start dancing around, don't be startled. "Don't give way to astonishment."

I'm a neurobiologist, so I'm interested in the brain. A lot has been written about DMT, and I'm not going to spend too much time talking about the experience. I think we're all aware of the nature of the DMT experience. This rather pithy quote is from Mr. [Graham] Hancock's book, where he describes the experience as "a highly artificial constructed inorganic and in essence technological kind of space."

The orthodox position with regard to the DMT state is to say, "Well, the DMT state is a hallucination." So my question is, Can we really explain the DMT state as mere hallucination? I expect that many of you in this room would say no, we can't, but that's not really good enough to just say that. As a neurobiologist I'm really interested in trying to understand: is it really possible to explain the DMT state as a hallucination? I will give you a heads-up now that I think the answer is no.

Let's assume that the DMT state is not a hallucination. The kind of model that has been propagated trying to explain it is what I call the tuning model, and many people have written about it. Certainly Graham has written about this idea that the brain is a kind of receiver; a receiver of *what* we will talk about, but one that can be tuned into this reality and under certain circumstances—perhaps precisely neurochemically defined states—it can also be tuned to another reality, rather like a radio. Sort of "Channel DMT" if you like. And I actually think that that's probably correct. But what I really want to understand and explain to you today is how that might work neurologically. What kind of mechanisms can we invoke that would explain how the brain can switch between channels? We'll start within a standard neurobiological paradigm, though we may need to transcend that and reconsider how we think about the nature of reality, and the way that reality is constructed, in order to explain DMT.

I'll start with a quote from the rather wonderful Hermann Hesse, which comes from his book *Demian,* a sort of semiautobiographical novel. "If the outside world fell in ruins, one of us would be capable of building it up again, for mountain and stream, tree and leaf, root and blossom, all that is shaped by nature lies modeled in us."

I think what's remarkable about that, other than the beautiful prose, is that this was written over a hundred years ago, or thereabouts, and yet it perfectly captures our current understanding of the way that our brain works in modeling the world. I'm going to be talking a lot about models today—models of reality.

The model of reality that we're all very familiar with is what's sometimes called the consensus model. Consensus reality, the reality that is largely agreed on. And the consensus model of reality is the standard model, by which all other models of reality are judged. Does your model of reality perfectly coincide with the consensus model of reality? It doesn't? Then it's not real. This is the standard by which we judge reality.

Some would say, "Well, that comes from evolution; this is biology—you can't argue with that," but I say even that's not the case. The brain cares not about truth. What I mean is that the brain's model of reality is the model that best allows it to make it to reproductive age and to reproduce. This is the basis of selection—fitness. That does not necessarily mean the model of reality must be the truest model of reality. Dennis [McKenna] on Tuesday said that the consensus reality is kind of a hallucination; it kind of corresponds to the real world. I would actually disagree—we have no way of knowing that. We have a functional, adaptive model of reality that best allows us to survive in whatever is out there, but there's no reason to think that this is the real thing, in any way.

In fact, people have looked at simulated worlds, with simulated beings, and examined whether it is always best for the sensory apparatus of the brain to model reality accurately. And actually that turns out not to be the case. Sometimes there are things that are excluded by the brain, ignored by the brain, or distorted by the brain. These things, for various reasons, will help you to survive in the world. So we can't simply assume that the consensus model of reality is the true model of reality.

So this is my axiom. I always have this in my presentations: "If a world appears to the consciousness, it must have an informational representation in the brain." What do I mean by informational representation? If you look around you the world is informative; everything around you is represented by information; the shapes of things, the positions of things in your field of view, the way things are moving, and the color of things; all of these must have a representation in the brain. You might disagree with that, and it might not be correct ultimately. But for example, if you have a stroke that affects the part of your brain that represents color, your world will become devoid of color. I suggest an experiment: give one of these stroke patients some DMT—will they see colorful visions or not? I suggest that they won't, but there's an interesting experiment if you disagree with me on this point.

So it doesn't matter whether we see a world as real or unreal. If a world appears to you, then it must have an informational representation in the brain. There's this sort of oft-quoted phrase or cliché: How do we define the difference between reality and unreality? If it's unreal, it's all in your head; and if it's real, it's not. But of course it doesn't matter whether it's real or not—the world must still have an informational representation in your brain. So I've barely started, and already we've dissolved the boundaries of what we can define as real or unreal. Which is the realest model of reality, and what's the difference between an unreal reality and a true one?

Hallucinations are often called false perceptions, and this is a definition you'll come across quite a lot, but we can never know whether a perception is truly false. We might perhaps call them—under certain circumstances—nonadaptive perceptions. But we cannot be definitive in deciding whether a perception is real or unreal.

So I'm going to talk about how the brain represents information. I already discussed what I mean by information: the way that your world is structured and constructed—not just visually, of course, as all the senses must be taken into account—is from information. What I tend to do is use a heuristic device, a simplified device, to explain and get you to understand what I'm doing. When you think of the part of the brain that is modeling the world, we're really talking about the cortex and particular areas of the cortex. The cortex is folded up inside your skull, but it's actually a flat sheet. We can imagine the cortex from a bird's-eye view, and it's broken up into these minimally functional units called columns, and these columns each have specific roles in representing information in the world. Of course, there are actually billions and billions of these columns, but if you can imagine a few from the side, then you would see that there are layers in these columns that are interconnected, and this is the basis for much of the computation in the cortex. But we're not going to get into that level of detail because it's not necessary.

What I will do is start by thinking about a really simple world or a simple object if you like. This is a very simple world that contains one object, such as a little alien face. When we look at this alien face it contains a lot of information. The position of the eyes, the shape of the eyes, the overall form of the head, and the mouth—this is all information and must all be represented in your cortex. So this is the visual percept if you like; this is what appears to your consciousness.

Let's now consider the representation in the brain. What I tend to use is a four-by-four grid of circles, where a circle is a column; so the grid is a representation of columns. And we can label functionally distinct areas: there's an area devoted to motion, an area devoted to color, an area devoted to form, and one for texture; by activating specific columns, you represent the informational structure of this little alien face.

In reality, of course, you have a very, very large number of these columns, billions of these columns, and they form these patterns of activation, and it's the patterns of activation that determine the structure of your world. This is how the informational structure of your world is represented. We can see this kind of rather complex pattern and notice that these columns are not independent. The world around you, although it is extremely informative, rich, and diverse and contains a range of different forms, colors, and shapes, is unified. And it is unified because these columns are interconnected. So rather than simply imagining it as a sort of mosaic of a pattern, you can see that it actually forms a unified structure because of these interconnections. Further, the connections aren't random or complete, but they also form patterns. They form a structure; we'll talk about what this structure means as we move forward.

This connectivity determines what's called the *intrinsic activity* of your cortical columns, which is the patterns of activation that your cortex normally adopts. In theory, your cortex could adopt a practically infinite number of different patterns, but of course not all of these would represent meaningful percepts; some of them would be completely meaningless. They certainly wouldn't represent an adaptive model of the world. So the brain has to sculpt the patterns of connectivity so that the activation patterns represent a useful model of the world. The connectivity allows certain patterns of activation.

Your brain is very good at building a world. In fact, your brain builds your world, your consensus model of reality, as a default. But the brain wasn't dropped to Earth, ready to start receiving data from this world and modeling it perfectly; it had to evolve the ability to do that. Although it's not completely understood how this happens, I guess the best way of thinking about it is to imagine that your brain is receiving this sensory data from the world that is activating specific populations of these cortical columns and strengthening and weakening the connections while also interacting with the environment. The patterns determined to be the most adaptive and functionally useful are selected for. It's called *neural Darwinism*. Again, we don't need to be bogged down in the details, but it's important that we understand that this ability to build this model of reality is something that your brain learned and evolved to do.

Another way to think about this connectivity is to imagine that all possible states that the cortical system can adopt are represented on a kind of attractor landscape, and only these low energy states are the states that are adopted. These are the states that build a representation of consensus reality that is functional, whereas the states higher up are inaccessible normally. As the brain evolves the ability to represent the world, a landscape is formed as the connections are molded and sculpted. This particular landscape develops until eventually you have this attractor landscape, this system of states that your brain adopts that represents consensus reality.

The brain is often thought of as a kind of camera that can take an image of the world. Actually, the brain must construct the world using this intrinsic activity that I've just explained. The brain uses very little—or far less information than you'd expect—to model this reality. Basically what happens is the small amounts of sensory data, or extrinsic information, are matched to this ongoing activity. The ongoing activity always provides the context for incoming data.

We can imagine some sort of informational pattern in the columns from the external world being matched to and amplifying specific patterns of activity that are always going on in your brain. So the brain really is tuned in to the types of sensory data that it receives from the consensus world.

A perfectly excellent validation of this model would be the dream state. When you are awake, the primary sensory areas of the brain that are receiving data or information from the external world are passing that on to higher areas that do most of the model building. But when you are asleep, these primary sensory areas are essentially cut off. That's not entirely true, but sensory data from the external world is largely excluded. During the dream state your brain is perfectly happy constructing the world. In fact the neural activity, this intrinsic activity, of the cortical system that builds the world in the waking state is exactly the same as in the dream state.

Researchers have looked at the amount of time you spend in a dream talking on a telephone or watching TV, and they actually find that this corresponds very well with the same proportion of time that you spend in the real world, in waking life. So dreaming really is, in its gross form, a continuation of waking. The difference between the dream state and the waking state is that the dream state is not modulated by this incoming sensory data, so this sensory matching is not going on—your world is being built entirely from this intrinsic activity. That still applies during the waking state, except extrinsic information is constraining and modulating the patterns that are adopted.

So the first take-home message is that the ability of the brain to represent any world—*any* world—must be learned, it must be evolved. This is an important point: your brain only knows how to build this world, or at least that's the way it should be.

Turning to psychedelic drugs, we can consider a columnar pattern representing the normal consensus reality state. As I said, the patterns of activation that model the world are restricted by this pattern of connectivity. For reasons that I'm not going to go into, when you introduce a drug like LSD or psilocybin, you get what I called in my 2013 paper a sort of "democratisation of the cortical columns," so the brain is able to adopt a larger repertoire of states. This is something I predicted in 2013, and then a year later Robin [Carhart-Harris]—whom we are very lucky to have here—and his team actually showed that this was in fact the case and that during the psychedelic state the brain adopts a larger repertoire of states. You can imagine what's going on is this attractor landscape is being flattened a little bit, so the brain can adopt states that it normally couldn't adopt. The world kind of moves; it shifts slightly from being very stable and predictable to being unstable, fluid, and novel.

But there's a bit of a problem in my opinion. When you introduce DMT into the brain, something different happens. It's not like the brain shifts from building the consensus world to building a slightly different version of the consensus world. It shifts, the channel switches, and it starts building a world that has no relationship whatsoever to the consensus world. With another kind of classical psychedelic like LSD, certainly at least at low doses, you get a novel activation pattern, yes. But when you introduce DMT, it's as if the brain is switched to a completely different mode, as if a different connectivity pattern has been adopted, such that the brain now builds with a beautifully effortless manner this extremely complex, extremely coherent, crystalline, beautiful, rich, and bizarre world that has no relationship to the consensus world. For me that's kind of confounding.

Another way you can think about it is rather than the attractor landscape being flattened, it's as if we shift into an entirely different attractor landscape.

We seem to have these two world-building modes that the brain has, depending on precisely defined neurochemical states and the interaction of specific receptor profiles. For simplicity's sake we can consider the 5-HT_{2A} and 5-HT_{1A} serotonin receptors, but others may be involved.

So the brain is shifting between these two world-building modes. Let's think about the consequence of that, using this model. Normally, in the consensus state this sensory data from the consensus world is matched to this ongoing intrinsic activity that is representing the consensus world. When you shift to the DMT state, sensory data from the consensus world no longer matches the activity of the consensus world. This is why when you smoke DMT—if you get a good dose— you don't generally go for a walk in the forest. You lie down, and you might even start screaming because your world is replaced. Data from this world, this consensus world, no longer matches this ongoing activity.

The question then becomes: Is the brain receiving data at all from another reality? We can imagine that as the activity of the brain changes, sensory data of a different kind that wouldn't have matched the ongoing activity earlier can suddenly be matched to this ongoing activity. So DMT alien data from this other reality can be matched. In other words, the brain acquires the ability to receive and render sensory data from another reality. So now we've got a neurological model for this switch. When serotonin is present, the brain adopts a particular pattern of activation that allows consensus data from this world to be matched, to be processed, and to be represented. But when DMT is present, you get this switch, so that consensus data no longer matches the ongoing activity, this data from this alternate reality. This is a neurological explanation for this previously rather vague idea of the tuning model, of switching between channels.

Earlier on, I said that the brain must learn to build; it must evolve the ability to build worlds, including the consensus world and, in my opinion, also the DMT world. When people smoke DMT, there is this remarkable sense of familiarity; people tend to go to the same kind of place, and the brain seems perfectly capable of building this kind of world. As we've shown, this ability must evolve, so you can imagine that the same process of neuroevolution—of how the brain learned to build the consensus world—can now be used to explain how the brain learned to build the DMT world. Instead of sensory data in the consensus world being sampled and modulating the connections, sensory data from the DMT world modulated those patterns of activation and developed a kind of parallel set of connectivities.

Of course, the problem with this is that it means that DMT must have been present in the brain for very long periods of time, and in fact there must have been periods when DMT essentially replaced serotonin. This is why I came up with this idea that DMT might be what I call an *ancestral neuromodulator*. DMT has a number of pharmacological peculiarities. It's an incredibly simple molecule—I sometimes call DMT a pharmacologically blunt instrument. All molecules have a set of structures that interact with the receptor, and the area where they interact is called a pharmacophore. DMT doesn't seem to have anchor points that anchor it into the receptor. In serotonin, you've got a hydroxyl group, which interacts with the receptor and is essential, and you also have the nitrogen. This nitrogen is still there in DMT, except it's masked by these other two methyl groups. Modeling studies have shown that this means the DMT nitrogen is actually unable to interact with the receptor. So it's very weird. If you were to look at that interaction not knowing anything about it, you'd say it is going to be inactive and is not going to do anything. But of course you'd be completely wrong about that. So DMT has these strange peculiarities and this curious affinity with the human brain that I think is difficult to understand.

So DMT is extremely simple. It's metabolized far more rapidly than other psychedelics, and it doesn't exhibit tolerance, which is unusual. As Dennis [McKenna] and Ede [Frecska] have spoken about, it's a substrate for various active transport systems in the brain. It has this very clean action—a clean switch from consensus reality to the DMT state. Perhaps there's a vestigial purpose? I'm using that word *vestigial* guardedly because it means that perhaps DMT doesn't have a modern function, but Ede is showing now that DMT possibly does have a modern function; but the levels in the brain are subpsychedelic.

If we think about our ancestry, our past, I developed this model of what I call parallel neural evolution, where I imagined that the brain cycled between serotonin production and DMT production. In the model, serotonin production peaked during the daylight hours—and that's actually the case, for example serotonin does drop when you enter the dream state—and then during the night time period, DMT replaced it. During daylight the brain would be interacting with this consensus world, and then during dreaming the brain would be interacting with the DMT world. I'm not saying here that DMT creates dreams. Dreams are very, very different from the DMT state. I'm actually saying that you would be having a DMT experience, and you would be interacting with the DMT world during this ancient form. Place it where you like in the past, in our evolutionary history—that's up for discussion. But the brain would be interacting with this DMT reality during the dream state. This raises a few interesting points because we now think, or many people think—although it's certainly not proven—that perhaps the pineal gland has something to do with DMT secretion. The pineal's modern function is to secrete melatonin, and this production is triggered by darkness. So it makes sense that as you descended into sleep at night, this darkness would trigger not just melatonin production but also perhaps DMT production.

I was reading Graham [Hancock's] book *Supernatural,* and in the early parts of the book he's talking about these caves, and inside them is Upper Paleolithic cave art depicting these strange creatures from beyond, and I think that Graham and others have suggested that this is because these individuals were having visions—they were shamans. It has always been assumed that they were ingesting some sort of drug. I suggest that perhaps this state was actually endogenous. I'd like to propose an ultimate explanation for why these paintings were done deep down in pitch-black caves, which is a very weird thing to do. But perhaps by going deep underground with no access at all to light, you would stimulate the pineal, which is stimulated by darkness and would produce endogenous DMT. By doing this, they would have DMT visions. Then you don't have to worry about where they got visionary plants, which ones they used, etcetera. But at some point in our past we seem to have lost this function and the ability to secrete DMT in psychedelic concentrations. Importantly, the brain still knows how to build this DMT world, because it learned to build this world a long time ago.

This also resonates with Tony Wright's idea that we have undergone an atrophication, a decline in neural function, in the past one hundred thousand years or so. One of the effects of this atrophication might actually have been a loss of this DMT-secreting ability, and we can also imagine the fact that, if we did have this ability, it might explain why we got ahead in the technological race. We could have been receiving data from this world in this early period. We had effectively been living parallel lives, interacting with this world during the daylight hours and interacting with this alien world when we were asleep during darkness. And we may have been receiving useful data in that regard. That's just an idea; make what you want of it.

So far we have established or suggested that the brain can switch between states: in one state it can receive data from this consensus world, and we know exactly how that works, and then during the DMT state it receives data from this alien world. Hopefully those of you who have been thinking would say this is a bit of a difficult question because we understand exactly how information from this world is sampled by the brain, but there doesn't seem to be a mechanism for the brain to receive data that doesn't come through the five senses, and DMT data certainly doesn't appear to come through the normal five-sense conduits. So how can the brain receive this kind of data?

This is really a bit of a problem. It's not the reality of this DMT world that is an issue—people always talk about whether the world is real. There's nothing in physics that says you can't have parallel universes populated with elves, or mantises, or other humanoids, or other strange creatures; there's nothing strange about that as such. What's remarkable, if this world exists, is that we can actually access it, because there seems to be no mechanism for data to be inputted. As we've seen, the brain must represent this world; the informational structure of the DMT world has to be represented in the brain. The question is, Is it being modulated by data from this DMT reality? If we say that DMT reality is truly a reality, then we need to think of a mechanism for how this data can be sampled.

In my opinion, that's going to require us to change the way that we normally think about reality. So far I've spoken about these activation patterns, but it's a kind of static structure. You can imagine these activation patterns shifting from moment to moment, representing each moment, each world, at each moment. But in fact the brain is an extremely dynamic structure, not only at the level of individual neurons, which undergo these complex oscillations and occasionally strange spiking activity, but especially when you get to large groups of neurons. Remember that the connectivity is the structure of the cortex, so groups of neurons adopt complex patterns of activity. But adding what we know from EEG, rather than thinking of the brain as representing information simply as a pattern of activation of these columns, it's better to think of the brain as more like an extremely complex vibrational structure composed of many different vibrational modes. This is what's called a *neural field model,* which treats the cortex as this unified structure.

If we consider the vibrational modes of a circular disk, it's the structure of the circular disk that determines the modes of vibration that it can adopt. Now that should ring a bell, because we said that the connectivity of the brain, which is its structure, determines the patterns of activity or the modes—the vibrational modes if you like—that it can adopt. That was our earlier model; it's a kind of static model, and sensory data is matched to this ongoing activity. Perhaps now we can change our model, or adapt it slightly to an equivalent model, and think of the brain as being this complex vibrational structure that is resonating with sensory data from the environment. This is completely equivalent to what I said before about sensory data being sampled, but I want to think about it slightly differently, as the brain—based on its structure and its connectivity—adopts this complex, vibrational mode that resonates with sensory data from the consensus world. The brain is tuned in to the consensus world rather like a bell; it's tuned in to a particular resonant frequency, for example. And in the same way, when you switch off the external source of the vibration, the brain, similar to a bell, continues to ring. This is what we're talking about in the dream state where the brain continues to represent the consensus world. In the dream state, the brain continues to ring, like a bell.

Now of course this also means that any information, from wherever, that does not resonate with this ongoing activity simply doesn't exist from the perspective of the brain. Earlier I said that during the consensus state, the normal waking state, DMT data could not be matched to this ongoing activity that generates the consensus world, so this DMT-state data doesn't exist from the perspective of the brain because it doesn't resonate. Of course, this works both ways. If you change the vibrational modes of the brain, perhaps using drugs, such that they no longer resonate with data from the consensus world, then the consensus world disappears; this is what happens during the DMT experience.

So far we've looked at two slightly different but really equivalent models of the way the brain models and samples data from the world. But if we want to explain the DMT state, we need to go a little bit further. We've really only been looking at the brain from the outside— what is the activity? Meanwhile all the interesting things are happening from within.

First of all, we really need to talk about what I consider to be one of the greatest mistakes in philosophy. I've spoken to a number of philosophers about this, and they generally blame René Descartes, but you might have different opinions. Basically, at some point in our history, we decided that we'd split the world into the subjective and the objective, what Pierre Teilhard de Chardin called the *within* of things and the *without* of things.

Now this caused many problems. It wasn't so much the splitting of reality into the objective and the subjective that was the problem; it was that for some reason we—although Descartes himself demonstrated that the only thing we can never deny is our own consciousness, our own mind—for some crazy reason we decided to regard the objective world that we can never get to as the ground of reality. Then we spent the next three or four hundred years trying to work out how this objective matter gives rise to this subjective world. We still haven't solved it, so we get all of these problems. Philosophers, particularly philosophers of mind, like to create problems for themselves and then spend a lot of time trying to solve them. The most famous of these problems is of course the *hard problem* of consciousness, which goes with the *easy problem* of consciousness, which is also quite hard.

We also have the *mind-body problem*: how does the mind relate to the body? Is it the same thing, all of this stuff? Ultimately, this really comes down to materialism and the idea that the world is constructed from matter, and somehow when matter is organized in certain ways it suddenly becomes conscious, which is very difficult to understand—hence the hard problem. But if we adapt, then the *hard problem* dissolves. For instance, we flip our model of reality and say, "Actually, there's no such thing as an objective world; everything is subjective, everything is constructed from consciousness"—and I'm sure many of you are sympathetic to that idea. We don't have to change our physics, by the way; just because we say that consciousness is fundamental doesn't mean that we have to consider consciousness to be this kind of amorphous field or soup. Consciousness has structure. Open your eyes, you can see the world around you; this is all consciousness, this has structure. We don't need to change our physics in any way; instead of regarding objective matter as being fundamental, we simply say that the subjective is fundamental. Consciousness is fundamental. The world is constructed from consciousness. This is really a form of idealism, but I'm not interested in 'isms here. When we do these things, the hard problem dissolves, because when we say that consciousness is fundamental we don't have to explain how dead matter becomes conscious. Also the *mind-body problem* goes away.

I think this is really where we need to be moving toward if we're going to explain the DMT state. We need to basically forget about the objective world. That doesn't mean that we're not interested in looking at brain activity, because that's really informative and it has been helping us so far, but we must understand that fundamentally everything is subjective.

This idea is perhaps quite difficult to get your head around, but I think it's really important that we do so. I highly recommend Bernardo Kastrup's book *Why Materialism Is Baloney*. He explains this model of reality rather better than I ever could: "If ever there was a perfect candidate to be sliced clean out of existence by Occam's razor, it ought to be the notion that an entire unprovable universe exists outside of mind." I think that puts it perfectly.

So what is a brain? Well, a brain is a structure that is formed from consciousness. It appears to be this kind of gelatinous structure from the outside. But if you imagine consciousness as not being this higher-dimensional structure, this matrix of consciousness, but rather imagine it as a one-dimensional line, you can then imagine that as this one-dimensional line folds up it forms knots, and these complex knots become self-reflective. So although consciousness is fundamental, there's also consciousness that seems to have this irresistible drive to self-complexify and self-organize. As consciousness forms these complex structures that we call brains, then these structures become self-reflective; so we are these foci, these points of view.

This way of looking at the world reminds me of the Hindu idea of Brahman, the fundamental ground of being, which some interpret as being consciousness, *Sat Chit Ananda,* "being consciousness bliss." Brahman plays at building the world. He doesn't do it because he needs to perfect himself—because he's already perfect, of course—but rather he is engaged in this thing called *Lila*: the game, the drama, playing at building the world. I think one way you can interpret Lila or the expression of Lila is that consciousness structured itself in such a way that it naturally self-organizes and self-complexifies to form these points of view. Then you imagine the self becoming lost in this world. Alan Watts described reality as this game of hide-and-seek, and that the self becomes many selves, with a small "s," and becomes lost in this world that it creates for itself. Well, how would you achieve that? By structuring yourself such that you naturally form these highly complex structures formed out of the matrix of consciousness, or Brahman, if you like, which then become many different individual points of view. So that, I think, is maybe a mechanism by which Brahman creates all the universe, including the DMT universe, of course.

Having changed this model of reality from the outside to the inside, we now need to change our model of what happens during the DMT state. So far we've looked at the brain from the outside and looked at its activity and tried to understand how it works, but now we need to move inward, because it's not so much the change in the structure in the activity of the brain that's important, it's actually the change in the structure and the activity of consciousness. We think about this same idea but from the subjective perspective. We've moved away from the brain. Now we're looking at the structure of the subjective consciousness.

The metaphor that's often used is the idea of a whirlpool in an ocean that has a certain structure, and that consciousness is this self-complexifying structure that forms this whirlpool that appears to be stable. It's actually relatively transient, but it seems to form this stable structure.

Earlier I introduced the idea of resonance to make it clear how we can think about consciousness as being a subjective structure, such that it resonates with the matrix of mind. And it's the structure of this self-reflective complex of consciousness that allows it to resonate with specific patterns in the mindfield, the infinite mindfield, or whatever you want to call it.

So what *we* are here is a group of these self-reflective complexes that occupy a collective reality. The reason we occupy a collective reality is because we all have brains, and we all have consciousness of basically the same type of structure, so we're all tuned in; we're all building a similar model of the world, therefore we're all seeing the world probably in a very similar way. We all adopt this consensus reality. So this is our collective reality—these little self-reflective complexes that have formed out of this matrix of mind.

If we try to think now about the larger structure of consciousness, this infinite matrix, I imagine that we are in a very small area of this infinite matrix of consciousness that is actually astonishingly complex, far more complex than we could possibly ever begin to understand.

So in this huge complex-consciousness matrix, these self-reflective complexes have formed, and they each occupy this collective reality. There could well be an infinite number. Importantly, wherever you get self-reflective complexes formed, they tend to have the same structure in the same area of this consciousness matrix, and they form a collective reality. We can imagine us being a separate collective reality. The only reason that they don't form a collective reality with other areas of the consciousness matrix is because their structure is different, so they don't resonate. These collective realities are completely separate. Distance isn't important. I'm not sure that distance is ever of any real significance, but it's really to do with this lack of resonant interaction.

So we've got a self-reflective complex that's formed somewhere in the matrix of mind. This could be an elf, for example, and it would be part of the collective reality of other elves and other DMT entities, which clearly are structured in such a way that they occupy their own collective reality. But of course as far as our collective reality is concerned, this elf reality doesn't exist because we are resonating with our particular structure in our area of the matrix of mind. So this DMT elf in his reality doesn't exist. But of course he does—and he's conscious! He's a self-reflective complex formed of consciousness. He is just as unable to deny his own existence as you are. But we can't communicate with him.

However, as we've seen, when you replace serotonin with DMT you get a change in the structure. We explain this in terms of the change in the patterns of connectivity and the change in the patterns of activation that can be adopted. You can think about this now as introducing DMT into consciousness, because we're moving to the subjective perspective. DMT causes the structure of consciousness to change such that its vibrational structure is altered and its vibrational modes are changed.

DMT changes the structure and the vibrational modes of this self-reflective complex. That means that this human with DMT present suddenly enters—not in a metaphorical sense but in a literal sense—the collective reality of these beings that before didn't exist. He leaves your collective reality. His body might appear to be still there, but that's just an image in your own consciousness; he is literally entering the collective reality of these beings, which are perfectly conscious.

Simply by changing our idea of reality slightly while still having our feet planted firmly in neurobiology, we can start to think about how we can communicate between these different collective realities, perhaps to get back important data.

In my opinion, I think we can take seriously the idea that these DMT entities are conscious, that they are aware of your presence, and may well be far more intelligent than you. So we need to open up an avenue of communication. We think of the DMT reality as another vibrational structure, another mode of the way that this consciousness tends to self-complexify and self-organize, and it's just as real as this one except normally we're unable to interact.

When we smoke DMT, we literally become part of the collective reality of the machine elves. I think we can perhaps think about alien abduction phenomena too. John Mack, toward the end of his life, moved away from the idea that these aliens were entering the bedroom physically and removing people from their bed; he thought they were somehow bringing these people into their reality. Perhaps they are using this method; perhaps they are from a different collective reality and were able to manipulate your neural structure, probably not using DMT. They probably have more efficient and rapid techniques to do that, but that could be an explanation.

I've recently become quite interested in simulated universe theory; the idea that this is a simulation by an advanced race of some sort, and the DMT state sometimes gives you the impression that perhaps they created us. They seem extremely intelligent, and you wonder perhaps did they create us and then embed DMT as this technology such that we can access and get the game? It's like a game, a cosmic game, a cosmic joke, in which the goal of the game is to work out that it's a game. And this is done through DMT, which you must discover. They place it everywhere in the environment, but you must reach the requisite level of cognitive sophistication to isolate it, understand it, and then work with it. Perhaps. I don't know.

But the reason I want to mention this is the idea that we need to start thinking about DMT as a technology, whatever its origin—whether it's an evolutionary origin or something that has been deliberately embedded. Now the usual way that DMT is ingested is by smoking. But of course the problem with this—and this is something actually that Rick Strassman spoke about yesterday—is that the effects are very short, they're very brief, so by the time you begin to even think about orienting yourself in this space you're already being dragged back. The reason for this is that when you administer DMT, whether by smoking it or by IV, or whatever, it floods the brain, but then it is metabolized and eliminated rather quickly, and you switch back to the consensus world.

This is a bit of a problem if we really want to use DMT as a technology. Some of you will say, well, you should drink ayahuasca. But as Dennis [McKenna] showed in his talk on Tuesday, when you drink ayahuasca, for a start the DMT levels never reach the same kind of concentrations as they do when you inject it or smoke it; it may be that you need to have a much higher level in the brain in order to completely flick the channel. Also of course with ayahuasca it's difficult to control the dosage; it's also associated with vomiting, and shitting yourself, and other unpleasantries that I'm told are very humbling. But if we want to treat DMT as a technology, we really need to use our technological sophistication and use it properly.

Now the problem with other psychedelics is that with repeated doses, you get some degree of tolerance. There are different types of tolerance and different mechanisms for tolerance. Again, they're not important; the important point is that with subsequent doses, the effect diminishes. Something that Rick discussed yesterday and demonstrated in his studies in the nineties is that even with repeated doses of DMT, you get the same effect every time. This is remarkable, but this makes DMT amenable to continuous intravenous infusion.

So I am suggesting something called *target-controlled continuous IV infusion* as the way that we could use DMT as a technology. If you go for an operation and the anesthetist wants to keep you asleep, what he doesn't do is just inject you with the anesthetic and then go home. He will often use this thing called target-controlled continuous IV that applies a mathematical model, which you get from pharmacokinetic studies, so that when the drug is injected into your body it then equilibrates with the various regions of your body. In the case of anesthetic, you are of course interested in its effects on the brain. By using this mathematical model you can control the administration over long periods of time, very carefully, so that you can maintain a stable brain concentration.

A skilled anesthesiologist can keep you in a state of anesthesia. He can bring you out of it slightly or he can push you slightly deeper during certain procedures. Importantly, he can maintain a very stable concentration; you don't want people waking up when you've got their chest cut open, and you don't want to give them too much such that they stop breathing; you want to maintain a stable concentration throughout the operation. We can use this very same technology that was developed for anesthetics with DMT.

I will justify this by talking about the requisite drug properties for target-controlled continuous intravenous infusion. The drug must have a rapid onset; it must have a short duration of action, so you don't get a buildup of active drug in the brain, which is very difficult to control. It must have a low-tolerance profile, and it must have a stable side-effect profile. DMT has all of these properties, making DMT a perfectly good candidate for target-controlled continuous IV infusion. What this means is that you can bring someone into the DMT state, and you might give them specific questions to ask, you might give them experiments to do, and you might even send a team of them all hooked up to this continuous IV machine; instead of being dragged back after a few minutes, they can spend time in the DMT space. In theory they can spend hours, days, weeks; you could even send them on a three-month vacation to the DMT world!

I will wrap it up there. I think we need to start using DMT in the way that the DMT entities would want us to. I think they want us to; they have lots to tell us, it seems, but we've so far been unable to bring back a lot of useful data. A part of this is because we haven't spent enough time there because of the way that we administer it. If we're going to learn, if we're going to open up two-way communication between these different collective realities, if we could validate the idea not only that these alternate dimensions exist but that we can actually communicate with them, then these would be the greatest discoveries in the history of mankind. Thank you.

DISCUSSION OF

The Neurobiology of Conscious Interaction with Alternate Realities and Their Inhabitants

BERNARD CARR: Andrew, I'm somewhat skeptical about these DMT intelligences, but I've been rather won over because there's such a striking similarity between the sort of model you've come up with, which is based on neurobiological grounds, and a picture that I briefly alluded to yesterday that comes from physics. So maybe I should just spend a minute clarifying what I mean about that.

ANDREW GALLIMORE: Please.

CARR: I explained yesterday how in modern physics you've got these extra dimensions, and I suggested that these extra dimensions could in principle be the arena of mental experience, the idea being that the physical world is just a slice, a four-dimensional space-time slice, of this higher dimensional structure. I think of that as a higher-dimensional reality structure. In fact, it's a sort of information space, and I personally regard that as a rather beautiful way of amalgamating matter and mind in a way that removes that artificial dichotomy that you refer to. But the point about this is that this higher-dimensional space is a sort of consensual reality; so one thing that I would slightly disagree with in your description is referring to *this* world [indicates room] as the consensual reality and the DMT world as something else. I would say in this picture that the DMT world is itself a consensual reality, but it's a different set of observers who are having the consensus.

GALLIMORE: Yes, yes.

CARR: Now the other interesting aspect of this model is that if you ask how these other dimensions are manifest, they actually correspond to essentially different levels of time and different experiences of time, which does effectively correspond to the idea that you can perceive this reality structure in different frequencies. So it really very neatly ties up with this idea that maybe the way the brain is receiving or accessing this other reality is through different frequencies. Which, I think, is what you were suggesting?

GALLIMORE: Yes, kind of, yes.

CARR: There's so much in your model. I loved your idea of the knots, because that idea corresponds very much with this concept of these consciousnesses as the nexus of connections in higher-dimensional space. And your beautiful simulation is actually exactly what happens—so I was really excited by that and especially since in some sense you're presenting a way of probing this experientially. Obviously, your last idea about having extended DMT trips is a great way of testing these sorts of models. Thank you very much.

VIMAL DARPAN: Thank you for your illuminating talk, Andrew. A couple of words about tolerance. I love the idea of the target-controlled IV infusion, and I think that could be a really amazing technology to definitively explore these realms. However, with regard to smoking DMT, there *is* actually a tolerance factor. If a good glass pipe of DMT is smoked, that's sufficient to break through fully into DMT space, and then another is smoked half an hour later, it's not quite as strong. There's a period that generally lasts about an hour when it is not so easy to get completely back in the zone.

GALLIMORE: This is important, and this is the kind of thing that needs to be looked at. There are different kinds of tolerance, and they might even be affected by the mode of administration that you're using. For all of these things, there is some mild tolerance, a low level of tolerance that can be accounted for in your IV model. Basically, in your pharmacokinetic model you can account for these factors. It's not a trivial thing. Rick [Strassman] mentioned this study in Germany that used continuous IV; they did use it, but they had a constant stream, and as long as the person was having an effect, they weren't modeling the level in the brain. So this is actually quite difficult and not a straightforward thing to do; you need really good pharmacokinetic and metabolic data.

DARPAN: Another thing is that given the fact that you don't have access to a target-controlled IV infusion apparatus or that particular technology, you might like to try three grams of *Peganum harmala* followed by smoking a full pipe of DMT . . .

GALLIMORE: No thanks.

DARPAN: . . . and it will extend the experience for a good hour. A good hour, but it's not for the faint of heart . . .

GALLIMORE: I'm not volunteering.

DARPAN: . . . deeply profound.

GALLIMORE: I will do the study, but I won't participate.

ROBIN CARHART-HARRIS: That was fascinating throughout, really, and I took copious notes. One thing that I found appealing—and you mentioned yesterday, which I need to think more about—is this idea that how consciousness is instantiated in the brain perhaps isn't so critical and that there's a way of understanding the phenomenology here without being so tightly bound to the study of brain activity. This idea of having weaker bounds between systems of the mind, let's say, rather than systems of the brain—systems that we associate with constructs like the ego and the phenomena of our unconscious mind—and that those bounds are weaker such that there is easier cross talk between those systems. So I found that really appealing.

Also, continuous infusion is something that we're looking to do at Imperial with brain imaging. And actually the tolerance idea is interesting because LSD and psilocybin typically last longer, and I wonder whether it's to do with the time at which a molecule is stimulating the receptor that determines tolerance. One thing, the thing that I wanted to question really, coming from the "greyer" perspective of being a strict—in my mind at least—scientist, was the idea that somehow the DMT state is separate from a psychedelic state and that it's an alien world that exists somehow. I don't know, I was getting a sense that [you were saying] it was almost separate from the brain or at least dependent on some kind of endogenous release of DMT. That just felt to me a bit of a leap, and I was going to suggest an alternative, you could say, a boring, perhaps more logical, perhaps less fantastical idea that the manifestation of these experiences actually arises from the intrinsic brain activity itself . . .

GALLIMORE: I'm going to pick you up there; that is exactly what I do say, that the DMT reality is the result of intrinsic activity of the brain, and the point I made is that all worlds that appear to consciousness result from intrinsic activity. The point is that the question is not whether the worlds—including the DMT world—are built from intrinsic activity, which they are. The question is, Is it modulated by this external data source? So all worlds that appear to consciousness are modulated and produced from this intrinsic activity. It's all in the head, always, but the difference between whether it's real or not, I guess, is more to do with whether it's being modulated by external sources . . .

CARHART-HARRIS: Can I fast forward to another question—whether there's any evidence for it?

GALLIMORE: [Pauses] Maybe someone can give you 50 milligrams in the brain, then come back to me.

CARHART-HARRIS: Yesterday somebody was talking about what these entities may have taught us, and I said, perhaps slightly naughtily, have they told us anything?

GALLIMORE: Yes, I know, I know, and this is why I'm suggesting we need to go in there for longer periods of time, and we can explore. As Dennis [McKenna] said, they must be explored in the usual way. I guess this is the usual way that we might do it.

CARHART-HARRIS: That boring alternative that I wanted to suggest was that the brain models the world, and there's a kind of chicken and egg relationship; it's formed by the world, and it also constructs the world in terms of our experience. But what happens in the psychedelic state is that there's a kind of anarchy in the system, there's a breakdown of bounds and separations, and there's a collapse of the normal hierarchical structure of the brain. For example, lower-level systems that are normally inhibited can have a kind of impetuosity to them, in that they can be anarchic in the way that they activate. So there is a kind of impetuous inference really, and models are called up. Classic models are iconic standards for certain images; for example, the brain thinks if entities exist, then they would likely have faces. It makes logical sense to me that the mind, the brain, will call up those models. It's logical that that would happen.

GALLIMORE: I guess the question is what are these models of reality? I'm not sure. The reason we're all interested in DMT is that it seems impossible, and yet the DMT world is undeniable; it cannot be denied once you've been there. And so I would dispute that we can say, "Well, it's simply these models that are overtaking the brain," in what you call this anarchic state. I think we can explain how the world becomes novel and fluid and unpredictable, and you might have illusions, and hallucinations, or whatever; but to jump from that and say the brain starts building these highly coherent crystalline worlds that are populated by astonishingly intelligent bizarre aliens, I think that's difficult to explain. And again, you need to smoke some DMT, dude.

[Audience laughter.]

CARHART-HARRIS: I think it's a much more fantastical leap—I think that's the point—and I would call it actually a wishful leap.

GALLIMORE: Okay, yes.

DAVID LUKE: We're going to have to go with the last couple of questions.

PETER MEYER: Can you go back to the issue of parallel evolution of night and day? How far back in our ancestry do you think that this parallel neuroevolution occurred? Is it prehuman?

GALLIMORE: I would say "I don't know" is the answer. I'm not an evolutionary biologist; perhaps Rupert will give a better answer to that. I would suggest that we're talking more than fifty thousand years ago, but I don't know.

MEYER: At which time humans have already evolved. But this might actually have occurred way back before humans.

GALLIMORE: Of course, it could have evolved way back before, but really, I think the better question is, When did we lose the function rather than when did we develop the function?

EDE FRECSKA: So you said that the information reaches only through the sensory organs, and we are resonating with the DMT entities. What is resonating? And which is coming through the sensory organs?

GALLIMORE: What do you mean, what is resonating—the receiver or the data source?

FRECSKA: You borrow the term from physics, and they say for vibration there is always a medium . . .

GALLIMORE: The medium is the structure. Remember that I spoke about the brain and the structure of the brain, meaning that it vibrates in a certain way that causes it to resonate with sensory data from the consensus world. But then I moved to the subjective model where I spoke about how it was the structure of consciousness that was vibrating and was resonating with appropriately resonant vibrational structures within surrounding consciousness.

FRECSKA: So you try to physicalize consciousness.

GALLIMORE: Well, I don't try physicalizing it . . .

FRECSKA: You denote it as a medium, a physical medium that vibrates.

GALLIMORE: The fundamental physical medium—I think that's reasonable to suggest. I think it's unreasonable to suggest that consciousness doesn't have structure. Of course consciousness has structure.

What I'm suggesting is that consciousness has properties that cause it to self-organize and self-complexify.

FRECSKA: You might as well say there's a green angel that resonates between us [laughs], between you and me.

LUKE: I'm afraid we really have to wrap this up, so I'm going to pass the last question to Erik.

ERIK DAVIS: To support Robin's alternative model, I would say that in your talk in general you didn't credit dreams enough. The dreams can be extraordinary. The dreams can be vibrant, technological, very fast, and full of beings. Clearly in your model, when we're shut off from any kind of external data, the brain has the capacity to produce extraordinary states. Not the same perhaps, not as vivid and with a different quality of presence, but with an extraordinary character. There are many dreamers who have extraordinary dreams that last for hours and involve multiple dimensions, technologies, and incredibly rich patterns that are greatly vivid. I've had a few DMT-inspired dreams that basically replicated the DMT state in the dream. That happened after I had been introduced to DMT, but it does show that a dreaming brain is capable of modeling extraordinary states.

GALLIMORE: I agree. I mean, the reason I spoke briefly about the dream state was really just to make the point that the brain is capable of building the consensus world even though it doesn't have any data and that during waking the only thing that's different really from a dream of the consensus world is that data is sampling and constraining the waking dream.

DAVIS: Okay, so I think you have to do more work to show how the novelty or the qualities of the DMT state are different enough that we cannot explain them in the same way we can explain in your model how vivid and novel dreams can be . . .

GALLIMORE: Yes, I agree, but I was limited by time.

DAVIS: I understand, but I think it's a real issue, because why can't we still invoke internal brain mechanisms of modeling? Another way of thinking about it is that you could imagine—and this is a speculation—that what DMT is able to do is get down to the engines of modeling. I won't go into a dream I had, but once I was in a dream world and I broke through the surface of the dream and I got to the sort of "dream machine" that was behind it, and the dream machine that was behind the dream was like the DMT state. To take that away from the metaphoric world of the dream, perhaps the capacity that the mind has to build worlds—it has little operators, little generators that produce three-dimensional objects—it's like you get down to the nitty gritty and it just grows intensely.

Now I'm not saying that that's more true than your proposal, but I didn't feel like you earned the "we can leave the internal-brain dream production, let's talk about an external reality" simply because it has the character of being realer than real—because of course that's also a mechanism that we have in the brain. It's impossible to answer this now, but I just wanted to say I very much appreciated the audacity and fascination of your presentation, but that was one part where I was not brought out of the "grey" world.

GALLIMORE: Okay. Thank you.

LUKE: We're going to have to wrap it up there, so thank you very much, Andrew.

CHAPTER 8

Morphic Resonance, Psychedelic Experience, and Collective Memory

Rupert Sheldrake

I think it's a very interesting time we are in at the moment, because there's a kind of transition of worldview that's going on that is being partly driven through psychedelic experience. So this is really cutting edge, and just now in Andrew [Gallimore]'s talk we fast-forwarded from brain-centered materialism, which only lasted about ten minutes, and then we were into quite other realms. So part of what we are in, in this room at the moment, is a kind of emulsion of different worldviews. But I think the transition that's happening at the moment is a move from materialism that has dominated science for more than a hundred years—the doctrine that all reality is material and that consciousness is nothing but a product of material activities in brains—to a view that includes a rediscovery of the idea of a *living* world, a living organic evolving cosmos, in which consciousness is both fundamental to the whole cosmos and reflected in many aspects of nature.

I think that we're moving beyond our cerebrocentric view of consciousness that tries to tie it just to brains and in some extreme cases just to *our* brains; more liberal materialists extend it to the brains of other animals but regard the rest of the universe as unconscious. I myself think that there's a kind of panpsychist aspect to nature. At all levels of nature there's a kind of mind, psyche, or some level of consciousness, even in electrons; that worldview gets interesting when you get to big things like the sun, stars, and galaxies—I think they're conscious too. So I think we live in a world full of consciousness, and I think that the basis of everything that happens is the ground level of being, the Primordial Mind, as Peter [Meyer] mentioned yesterday. I think we're in the presence of a greater consciousness all the time.

What I'm going to do to start is talk about morphic resonance, because this is one way of looking at things differently. It's part of the shift from the materialist view to a more organic view of nature. Morphic resonance is basically the idea that there's a memory inherent in nature and that the so-called laws of nature are more like habits. All species have collective memories, where each individual draws on the collective memory and in turn contributes to it.

The basic idea of morphic resonance is that similar self-organizing patterns of activity resonate with previous similar patterns of activity, across space and time. Now if you say, "What's the mechanism?" then my answer is, I don't know. There's a variety of hypotheses as to how this could happen—multidimensional realities, implicate order, extensions of quantum theory—but anyway the postulate, the hypothesis, is this is how nature works.

When I first thought of this idea I was a don [professor] at Cambridge, and when I discussed it with my colleagues on high table [the formal dinner table for academics] and in the biochemistry department tea room, I didn't find a very warm reception to this idea; in fact, most people couldn't understand what I was trying to say. I then took up a job working as an agricultural scientist in India, and I found an exactly opposite response. When I mentioned this idea to my colleagues there, most of them, the Hindu ones especially, said, "Oh there is nothing new in this idea, ancient rishis have said this thousands of years ago." In Hindu and in Buddhist philosophy the idea that there's a kind of memory in nature is totally mainstream, known to virtually everybody. I'd meet random people on trains—and in India they all like to interact on these long train journeys—they ask you first your name, then where are you from, and then how many children you have, then what your salary is [laughter]. And after they've done the basic questions, then they say, "What is your view of the universe?" So you get into these conversations, and I had many; so I thought, okay, well, I'll bring in morphic resonance, and almost everyone had this reaction: "Oh, what's so new about this . . ."

It's interesting, you see, that something so shocking in the West is so normal in the East, and I found it really encouraging that seemingly sane people thought this way and had done so for a long time. I wrote my first book when I was living in India. Anyway, the idea is testable and leads to a lot of possible experimental tests, some of which have already been done. It applies to crystals as well as living organisms and to molecules. The hypothesis says that if you crystallize something for the first time, that if a crystal's never been made before, it would be hard to crystallize, to wait for a new form to come into being in nature; but next time you do it it'll get easier, and the third, fourth, and fifth times get easier and easier because of morphic resonance from previous crystals.

If you train rats to learn a new trick in one place, then rats all over the world should be able to learn the same thing quicker, because the rats have learned it somewhere else in the world. So there's a kind of memory in nature. There's been quite a few tests, and they're summarized in the new edition of my book *A New Science of Life*, third edition [2009]. I'm not going to go into the empirical evidence now, I'm just going to say that it's a hypothesis. I should also say, because it's not obvious, that it's a controversial hypothesis. I'll explore some aspects of it and show how they might relate to psychedelic experience.

First of all, morphic resonance leads to a new view of inheritance. A lot of the form and instincts of animals and the forms of plants are inherited by morphic resonance—not by genes—so I've been saying for years and years that genes are grossly overrated. I think what they do is what we know they do: they code for the sequence of amino acids and proteins, but they don't code for the shape of your face, or for an orchid flower, or for the web-spinning instincts of a spider. Those kinds of things are inherited by morphic resonance, not from genes. The concept of the genetic program is an attempt to explain how genes could lead to the inheritance of things like this, but it's a metaphor, and it's not a very good metaphor. Genes don't do most of the things they're supposed to do, and this has now become widely recognized.

In the past three or four years within biology there has been a crisis, which goes under the name "the missing heritability problem." By sequencing tens of thousands of genomes of different people, attempts to identify genes for height, cancer proneness, and lots of other characteristics have been extraordinarily unsuccessful. They lead to a predictive value of genes—knowing a great deal more about genes than anyone's ever known before—of about 5 to 10 percent, and this is for characteristics that are known to be 80 percent heritable. So the gap between the 5 percent the genes explain and the 80 percent that's inherited—the 75 percent that's missing—is called the missing heritability problem.

I think that's because genes just can't and don't do all the things that people used to think they did. This is now very much an issue within biology; the old genetic model is coming unraveled, and the evolutionary model based on selfish genes and random mutation, the neo-Darwinian model, is also coming unraveled because of the recognition of epigenetics.* The biggest taboo of twentieth-century biology is now mainstream. It's been rebranded, and this in turn has thrown evolutionary theory into turmoil because if organisms can inherit things their parents learned or forms that they adapted or acquired in just a single generation, then neo-Darwinism seems highly inadequate; as a kind of

---

*Epigenetics is the inheritance of acquired characteristics.

creativity goes back into living organisms, it's not just random chance. These are all issues that journals like *Nature* are full of at the moment. There was a big debate in the past two or three months on the need for an extended evolutionary synthesis that goes beyond neo-Darwinism.

So I think morphic resonance underlies the inheritance of form and of instincts and also enables things that have been learned to spread within populations much more quickly than they would normally spread. Because it depends on similarity, you'd expect it to happen most between organisms that are the most similar, like identical twins; indeed, there do seem to be many similarities between identical twins, even those who were separated soon after birth. These are normally taken to say, "Well, it's all in the genes," but actually I think the evidence is much better explained by resonance between the twins.

The bit that becomes quite relevant to our concerns here is when we think about who's the most similar or very similar to you in the past, and the answer is you. We're more similar to ourselves in the past than to anyone else, and that means the most specific resonance working on us from the past is from our own past. In other words, I'm suggesting our memories may not be stored in our brains but rather depend on morphic resonance. The brain is like a tuning device, a receiver, but it's more like a TV set than a video recorder. So I think memories depend on brain activity. When memories are being laid down, you can actually measure activity in the brain, in the hippocampus and other regions, and when they're being retrieved you can also measure activity in the brain. But I think that in between they're not stored inside the brain; I think the brain is a kind of resonating system that can tune in to them. Attempts to locate long-term memory traces have been remarkably unsuccessful, and I think that's because they're not there. But this is a paradigm, you see, a model of reality within neuroscience. It's just taken for granted they must be in the brain because where else could they be?

Now as soon as we think like this we recognize that the collective memory is also an important part of our experience. Jung put forward the idea of the collective unconscious and collective memory, but it didn't fit with contemporary genetic theories at the time, so it wasn't taken very seriously. But it is a concept that would have to be invented if it didn't already exist. I think we all tune in to a kind of collective memory.

This becomes relevant if we think about what's going on with different kinds of psychedelic experience. If you take a substance like mushrooms, or DMT, or ayahuasca, this has physiological effects on the brain: certain changes in brain activity, differences in the membranes, and all kinds of molecular mechanisms have been worked out. Those happen in a similar way in different people's brains, so if I take a substance, my brain's put into a special state that's associated with having that substance, and my experience will involve tuning in to people who've taken that substance before. Each of these drugs will have its own kind of collective memory, a pool of experience from those who've taken it before. And in the case where drugs have been taken in shamanic cultures, then the whole field of that experience will be heavily charged with the elements from that culture.

There was a very interesting study by Claudio Naranjo that some of you are probably familiar with, where he gave ayahuasca to people living in urban settings in South America. These were middle-class people who knew nothing about tribal cultures, and they started having visions full of jaguars and all sorts of other elements that come from the cultures in which these substances had been used psychedelically. It looked as if people were tapping into a kind of memory. Well, there are two hypotheses: one, you could say these molecules activate cells in the brain that produce jaguar imagery through some kind of molecular mechanism—which doesn't sound very likely—or two, that you're tapping into a kind of collective memory.

I discussed this with Sasha Shulgin and Terence McKenna at a gathering of about this size at Esalen [California]. There were two or three gatherings that Jill [Purce] and I went to at Esalen in the 1980s, called ARUPA conferences. ARUPA is the Association for the Responsible Use of Psychoactive Agents. I like to think of experiments, so I tried to create a way to test the collective memory psychedelic theory. I needed someone who created new drugs; Shulgin did that all the time—he was the ultimate designer of designer drugs. I asked him what it was like when he first took a drug that he'd synthesized that no one had ever taken before. And he said that he always took it himself first, and then if it wasn't toxic and so on, he would have a tasting panel of about twelve people take these drugs. Then they'd compare notes, and a consensus emerged about what the drug did. No one knew before a consensus emerged. Then as more people took it, this consensus grew.

It seemed to me that one could change the consensus reality by having the drug taken under particular conditions; so you'd have, for example, six possible settings in which it could be done—Japanese themed, psychedelic art themed, outdoor English garden themed, etcetera—and for all the first people who took the drug, you'd pick at random one of these settings. You'd throw the die to determine whether it was Japanese or English garden, then the first dozen or two of people who took it would take it within that setting, say, an English garden. Then you'd have people from other places in the world take it, and if everyone started getting English-garden imagery, then it would rather confirm the morphic resonance theory. Anyway, no one's actually done this experiment, but in principle it's possible to test it.

Morphic resonance also means that we can see rituals in a new way. All relations, all social groups, have rituals. Rituals very often reenact the primal story of that group. For example, Jewish people have Passover every year, which reenacts the original Passover dinner in Egypt as they left to go through the wilderness to the promised land, and the Christian Holy Communion, itself a Passover meal, reenacts the last supper of Jesus with his disciples. The American Thanksgiving dinner reenacts the first thanksgiving of the settlers in the New World and so on.

All rituals tend to be conservative, and people feel that they have to do them the right way by using the right language, making the right food, and creating the right smells. Many liturgical languages are highly conservative too; the Coptic Church in Egypt still uses the only surviving forms of the ancient Egyptian language in its liturgy. The Russian church is in old Slavic; in the English church many people prefer the Elizabethan form of language to the modern one. So there's this conservative element to rituals. I think one reason for this is that if things are done in as similar a way as possible to the way they were done before, then there's a resonance between those who are doing it now and those who'd done it before, a presence of the past, a connection with those who'd gone before. That's what most people doing rituals think they're doing; they think they're reconnecting with those who did it in the first place and all those who've done it since over the generations. It's a connection across time. In tribal cultures this connection across time is taken for granted as a key part of the whole culture. In our world, which is rather more ahistorical, most people think that society is just the living, but almost all traditional views of society include the ancestors as well as the descendants, and through rituals we're linked to the whole tradition in which we grow up and live.

I think that some kinds of rituals and rites of passage are of great interest here, because I think some rites of passage involve dying and being reborn. Some of them do it symbolically; I think some do it literally. Near-death experience is something that has been quite widely studied in the modern world, partly because there are more than ever before; far more people get resuscitated than they ever did in the past, so there's more opportunity to observe near-death experiences. Near-death experiences involve a variety of events. Not everyone has them, but those who do often find themselves floating above their body and going through a tunnel into a realm of light where they meet beings, ancestors, or other entities. This kind of near-death experience—which means people say they've died and they've been born again, they've gone beyond death, and they're no longer afraid of death—changes people's lives.

I think in many traditions these have actually been induced deliberately. In the Christian tradition, I think this is what happens through baptism. I think John the Baptist held those being baptized under the water just long enough; in the space of two or three minutes you could hold someone under just long enough to induce death by drowning—their life would flash before them, they could leave their body, and they'd see themselves from outside. They'd come back, and when they were revived on the bank of the Jordan they'd say they'd died and been born again and that their life was transformed; that's exactly what they said, and I think that's exactly what was happening. There's no reason to suppose this was just symbolic. Why do it symbolically when you can actually do it literally? Of course, John the Baptist had the big advantage of operating in the days before litigation.

[Audience laughter.]

ANTON BILTON: Rupert, not so; he ended up with his head on a plate . . .

SHELDRAKE: That's true, he came to a sticky end, but that wasn't because of liability litigation. When adult baptism was revived by the Anabaptists in the sixteenth and seventeenth centuries, they reinstated baptism by total immersion, and of course it's the Baptists, particularly in America the southern Baptists, who go on most about dying and being born again—born-again Christians. They actually sought out baptism by total immersion. Now, America is of course full of litigation, so probably not many of them do it for very long, but I myself think that in the sixteenth and seventeenth centuries they probably did it seriously, and that this was a real experience for people.

Now of course a near-death experience is by definition one from which people haven't actually died; they've come back again. There have been a lot of studies on near-death experiences that show brains flatlining during the actual experience, so it's hard to say, "Well, all of this experience is correlated with this kind of brain activity." They're flatlined because they measure the EEG in cardiology operations and show that there's actually no brain activity measurable through the EEG.

These experiences are being much studied, and I think they're related to rituals. Many people who've taken DMT feel that they've had a near-death type experience. The first time I took it, I myself had this experience that involved breaking through a tunnel into another realm of light, and I didn't encounter all these beings we've been hearing about, but I did encounter a feeling of being in a state of total bliss, in what seemed to me like divine consciousness.

This near-death-like quality of this experience was so striking to me that I got very interested in discussing that aspect of it. I do think, in fact, that one of the things that is happening in some of these DMT experiences is something very like a near-death experience, and it may be that by morphic resonance we're actually tuning in to people who have had near-death experiences. Near-death experiences, as I say, usually involve encountering other beings. People have the feeling they're being welcomed by people on the other side. So that doesn't explain the experience itself, but it does explain how certain elements of it could resonate with them through a kind of collective memory in these DMT trips.

I want to turn now to the question of survival of bodily death, because this is something that's also relevant to interpreting these experiences, and any discussion of survival of bodily death has to deal with the question of memory. All theories of survival require the survival of memory. Theories of reincarnation require habits or dispositions, in some cases explicit memories, to be carried over from one life to another. Usually in the cases that Ian Stevenson studied it was children who remembered previous lives, involving quite a lot of explicit memory. Believers in reincarnation say, "Well, usually we don't remember the details; it's just the habits or dispositions that are carried from life to life." Nevertheless, there has to be some kind of transfer of memory; otherwise the concept of reincarnation becomes meaningless, because it's not the physical person that's reincarnated, it's the mind with the memories.

The traditional Western theory, in the Catholic tradition, is of purgatory, where after you die there's a continued period of development.

You still go on roughly like you do in this life to start with, but you can continue to develop until you're ready to go beyond the more limited state into a state of fusion with divine consciousness, or bliss. So there's an ongoing development, but that again requires memory. Extreme Protestant theories of survival—which say you go to sleep when you die, you're woken up by a trumpet for the last judgment, and you appear before your maker to be judged—require memory too, because if you appear before your maker and you've forgotten who you are and what you've done, then it wouldn't be a very meaningful experience.

When I was an atheist, I used to like the idea of memories being stored in the brain because it was so easy to confound believers. You'd say to them, "Do you think you survive bodily death?" And they'd say, "Yes," and you say, "Do you think you'd have some kind of memory?" They'd say, "Yes." "So what do you think happens to your brain when you die?" and they'd say, "Well, it breaks down." "So where are your memories stored?" And they'd say, "Well, in the brain." So they were instantly floundering.

But the thing is, it does depend on the assumption that memories are in the brain. If memories are not inside the brain, then they're not necessarily destroyed by death. We may normally need our brain to tune in to our memories, but if the memories are not stored in the brain, then it's possible for memories to survive the death of the body, and this opens the way to a variety of theories of survival. The conventional theory, the materialist theory, closes the door on all conceivable religious theories of survival, just slams the door closed on the basis of dogmatic assumption. If memories are not in the brain, as I think they're not, then it leaves the door open for all sorts of possible forms of survival to be considered.

My own view is that when we die, after a kind of near-death-type experience, we enter a kind of dreamlike state. Basically, I think when we die we can go on dreaming, but we can no longer wake up, because we haven't got a physical body to wake up in. We're trapped in a kind of dream realm. Now, all of us have dream bodies. Every night when you dream you have a body in your dreams that is different from your physical body: you can move around in it, you can talk to people, you can meet other people, you encounter beings in your dreams, and animals. And they've got bodies too. You're not necessarily looking down to check that your body's there in your dream, but you have a center of consciousness that moves around. Most of the time I'm not checking that my body's here; I just take it for granted as a center of consciousness. That's what we have in our dreams.

I think that if when we survive we go into a kind of dream state, then this is completely democratic because it allows everyone to have exactly what they expect. If you're a suicide bomber and you think you'll end up in an oasis with almond-eyed dancing girls serving you dates, you may well get that for a while. If you're an atheist and you think everything goes blank, that's perhaps what'll happen. And what happens to you depends on your expectations, your beliefs, your experiences, your hopes, and so forth. If you pray and meditate when you're alive—and you can go on doing that in a kind of dreamlike state after death—then there's a possibility of spiritual development and liberation from this dreamlike world. This is essentially a version of purgatory theory that I'm putting forward.

So in our dreams, in our dream world when we're alive, we have a dream body. We encounter other beings, and some of those beings that we encounter are dead people. I sometimes meet people in my dreams I know have died. Are they just figments of my imagination, or is there a dream world in which all dreamers have some grounds of overlap? Some people living in close communities share dreams. Some of our dreams may be highly individualistic or idiosyncratic; other elements may be shared, and there may be real opportunities to meet other beings, including people who are dead, in our dreams. In the Old Testament there are many stories of visions of angels and beings in dreams that are taken very seriously by the prophets. This is one of the things that Rick Strassman has written about in his recent book on DMT and the spirit of prophecy. So here we have a realm of beings, the deceased, which

could include dreamlike bodies or people in dreamlike states, interacting with other deceased people in dreamlike states. Whether or not
this realm includes similar dreamlike bodies of animals that have died I
don't know. I don't see why not; many animals dream too and probably
must have dream bodies. When a dog is dreaming of running along,
you can see from its legs twitching that it's dreaming and presumably
dreaming about chasing a rabbit or a ball or something. It has a dream
body; maybe there are countless dream bodies of animals in this realm
as well.

Then there's a whole realm of beings. Most traditions have admitted
spirit beings of various kinds; in the Western tradition they're angels.
The study of angels, or angelology, is not something that's much taken
up today, and you can't get degrees in angelology from most universities.
I became very interested in this a number of years ago with a theologian friend, Matthew Fox, and we decided to investigate the traditional
Western angelology. We read the books on the subject by Dionysius
the Areopagite [now called Pseudo-Dionysius the Areopagite], a sixth-
century Syrian monk who was much influenced by the neo-Platonic
tradition, of which Peter [Meyer] told us something yesterday. Also,
we read Hildegarde of Bingen, a medieval visionary abbess in Germany
who saw angels, and St. Thomas Aquinas, the great synthetic mind of
the Middle Ages who in his *Summa Theologia* has an entire two books
on angels, *De Angelis*. We read all these texts, made an anthology of
the most interesting passages, and then had a dialogue on each passage.
That's all printed in our book *The Physics of Angels*.

The reason it's called *The Physics of Angels* is that when I was
reading Aquinas, I was very struck by his description of these beings.
Aquinas had an extraordinarily clear mind, and when he's discussing
how angels act, he says: "We know them through their actions, when
an angel acts somewhere, it acts in a place because they have to be
located to act in the physical world. And if it can act in one place,
they can move from one place to another." So he has an entire section
where he discusses the movement of angels. And in the movement of

angels, he says the angel must act with its whole being when it acts. In other words they're quantized: each angel is a quantum of angelic action, and you can't have half an angel acting; you have the whole angel acting. And when they move from one place to another, from the point of view of an external observer, time would elapse, because the angel is moving, and it can't move at infinite speed. From the point of view of the angel itself, however, no time elapses when it moves from one place to another. It's exactly what Einstein thought about photons: he said from the photon's point of view no time elapses, but from our external point of view eight minutes elapses for it to get from the sun to the Earth. Anyway, I was very intrigued by the parallels between angels and photons in Aquinas; that was how we came up with the title *The Physics of Angels*.

Angels are central and mainstream in Judaism, Christianity, and Islam. In India they have the *devas,* or great realms of beings, and the Tibetans have *dakinis.* Almost all traditions have the idea of innumerable beings. Their nature is obscure—of course, they're not as depicted in stained-glass windows, good-looking and slightly epicene humans with colored wings—and nowhere in Aquinas or Hildegarde does any description of angels look remotely like what most people today would describe them as. They were iconographically pictured like they appear in Sumeria, where they had winged beings. In Ancient Greece, they had winged beings symbolizing the power to move from one place to another with freedom—I think this is rather like in dreams. If you have a lucid dream you can move from one place to another as if you're flying.

So there is this whole realm of beings in this tradition of angels—and you may think this is not very relevant to modern biology, but it's curiously relevant in one way that's not often appreciated. We know that Alfred Russel Wallace coinvented evolutionary theory with Charles Darwin; both of them came up with the idea of evolution by natural selection. Wallace was one of the great pioneers of evolutionary theory, but we hear a great deal more about Darwin's gloomy views about evolution being purposeless and so on, and we hear much less about Wallace's views on evolution. In his last book, *The World of Life* published in 1911, Wallace puts forth the idea that the innovation and creativity in evolution can't possibly be explained by just blind spontaneous variation with no creativity or intelligence. He thought that the evolution of the different levels of beings—cells, tissues, organs, and the many different kinds of plants and animals—was guided by intelligent spirits, which he considered to be angels.

So Wallace's theory of evolution is that it's guided by angels. It's interesting that he thought that there were these beings. In light of our discussions here, it just occurred to me yesterday that Wallace spent years in the Amazon, and his first studies were traveling in remote parts of the Amazon as an explorer. He then went to the Dutch East Indies, to Flores, and to various parts of what's now Indonesia. But during his formative years, when Darwin was going around on the *Beagle* and just dipped into South America from the ship, Wallace was spending years immersed in explorations of the Amazon. Did Wallace take ayahuasca? is the question that sprang to my mind; his idea of these beings guiding evolution would take on a completely different complexion if he had. He was certainly an explorer; Terence McKenna regarded him as his role model for exploring with a pith helmet, in the usual way, but Wallace may have been more of a role model than even Terence thought.

There's a field that I myself am very interested in, which I find hardly anyone else is interested in outside the narrow professional group; namely, theology. State-of-the-art theology today is extremely interesting, and I think it is one of the more fascinating areas of consciousness studies. Old-style theology from the seventeenth century onward tried to adapt to the mechanistic worldview. They said, okay, the world's a machine, God's an engineer who made the machine; you've got the idea of God as an intelligent designer, designing the machinery of nature and then intervening, suspending the laws of nature to intervene in the working of nature. This is a view of God that atheists don't believe in, and I don't believe in either. I'm not an atheist, but I think it's a completely incredible view of God.

What's been going on in theology in the past twenty years is a rediscovery of pre-seventeenth-century Christian theology, which was much influenced by thought from other parts of the world and is grounded in views of consciousness that are very well summarized in a recent book. The state-of-the-art book on modern theology is called *The Experience of God: Being, Consciousness, Bliss* by David Bentley Hart, who is an American theologian and Greek Orthodox by faith. What he shows is that traditional views of divine consciousness have far more in common among traditions than what separates them, and there are very great similarities among Hindu views, Christian views, Sufi views, and views in other traditions as well. The subtitle of his book, *Being, Consciousness, Bliss,* reflects the Hindu model of ultimate reality, Sat Chit Ananda, to which Andrew [Bilton] referred.

Basically, the traditional view is that the ultimate ground of being from which all things come and from which all forms of consciousness arise is the being of God, which sustains the universe from moment to moment; that's why we're here now, sustained from moment to moment. God is not a remote demiurge that starts things off at the beginning, but rather God is the sustainer of all being at all times. Consciousness is to do with forms and knowledge and so on. In the Christian model of this it's the *Logos,* the formative principle, the word principle. And then the spirit, in the Christian tradition the Holy Spirit, is the movement of energy through the universe. And within the being of God this energy takes the form of bliss, because God's consciousness is within an eternal present; therefore in any contact with the divine consciousness through mystical experience, there is an experience of being, knowledge, and bliss. This is direct contact with divine consciousness. God is known not through studying the external world to see if you can find God in outer space or something, but rather God is known through the exploration of consciousness. God is a conscious being who's known through consciousness.

That's the basic foundation of the religious traditions of East and West. The primary knowledge of God is through direct experience. The distillate of this is that the divine has these three aspects: being, consciousness, bliss. The Christian version, the Holy Trinity, is based on metaphor of speech and, in the primary metaphor, the word and the spirit. God the father is the speaker and the ground of all being, and the metaphor is that the Word forms patterned structures—they're vibratory patterns of activity, words with meaning, interconnection, and so on. But words can only exist in the world if they're carried by the breath. As I'm speaking now there's an outflow of breath; if I don't have that outflow of breath that carries my words through the air to you, then they're silent inside my mind, and they do nothing. But to be expressed in the world you have to have a flow of energy, and you also have to have a form, pattern, or structure; the two together are vibratory patterns.

This is the basic model of the divine nature, and in medieval theology the idea was that all plants, all animals, and all beings reflect this divine nature. In modern science we'd say that the field aspect of things—fields are what give form structure, pattern, and order; and energy is what gives flow, change, movement, and activity—is reflected in all beings. Saint Bonaventure, who was a Franciscan in the thirteenth century, thought that all beings reflect the trinity in the divine nature. The pope's recent encyclical *Laudato si'*, on the environment, is a fascinating document based entirely on the Franciscan vision of living nature, in which we're part of the living world, we're part of nature. Nature is in God, God is in nature. It's a panentheistic God-in-nature, nature-in-God view. It's based very strongly on St. Francis of Assisi, and after all, Pope Francis took St. Francis's name when he became pope. The opening words of the encyclical *Laudato si'* are a quotation from St. Francis of Assisi. It's very fascinating that this, what some call neo-orthodox theology, now permeates the Vatican; there's no mention of a kind of world with God as an external machine maker, designing the machinery of nature. Rather, this is a view of living nature filled with consciousness and reflecting divine consciousness throughout.

Now, I myself think that the way in which some psychedelics act is through disturbing normal neurotransmitters and normal brain activity, releasing us from the direct connection with sensory reality; that's what happens in our dreams, as several people have mentioned. I think that a drug like DMT—which in high doses stops us from doing anything, you're sort of paralyzed by it, really—liberates us from the normal constraints on our mental activity, just as dreams are liberated from the normal constraints of sensory inputs. Other psychedelics can disturb normal patterns of activity, allowing this immense capacity for forming images and worlds that we experience through our dreams. I think they open up these realms of consciousness.

I myself think that in the near-death-type experiences with DMT and in blissful states induced by other drugs, we are actually linking to the divine mind. I think mystical experiences are not, as materialists would say, just produced inside the brain through short-circuiting bits of the brain and through molecules affecting axons, neurons, synapses, and things. The potential to participate in the divine mind is there all the time—but normally we block it out. In the Dzogchen tradition and in Krishnamurti's teachings, the idea is it's here now, all the time, it's just that we block out access to it, we create barriers; because we're so busy getting on with our normal lives, and with all the distractions that the modern world has to offer, it's probably more blocked out in our civilization than in any previous one. But there is this potential for contact with the divine mind, and psychedelics are one way in which this can happen.

So I think that if we're talking about the nature of consciousness, any big-scale view has to take into account divine consciousness as well as the consciousness of the sun and the galaxies and many other forms of organization in nature. Just focusing on the brain is much, much too narrow; it plays an important part, but the big picture, I think, has to include theology, or if you like philosophy, old-style philosophy of ultimate reality. Otherwise we have too incomplete a view of consciousness, and in understanding our own explorations, we can't see the big picture within which we're operating.

In conclusion, I think that the psychedelic revolution—the expanding interest in psychedelics—is one of the things that's actually driving the paradigm shift at the moment, because most people aren't very interested in reading detailed arguments about the nature of reality, the nature of nature, and so forth. I am personally, but I very soon realized that this is a minority interest, whereas most people are interested in their own experience—and rightly so. If they've had experiences that break open their worldview and show that it is far too limited, far too incomplete, then this breakthrough is a very important part of a quest for something else.

The temple here [at Tyringham Hall] has an inscription about being in the quest; is it the quest for truth? Normally, most people don't feel much motivation to go on a quest to a truth—life's too full of distractions and answering emails and things—but psychedelics do inspire such a quest. They did for me. My first experience was with LSD in 1971, and it completely changed my view of reality. I think for many young people now psychedelics are a rite of passage; they're like a near-death experience, like dying and being born again into a new world and a new reality. I think that what we're talking about here is actually at the cutting edge of this transition in our culture, because most people change their worldview because of experience; and it's now on a mass scale that people are taking psychedelics, often unwisely, not well guided, and there are casualties along the way; nevertheless, I think it's an extraordinarily powerful driver of this change. It's not really coordinated or organized by anybody, it's just happening, and that's why I think that what we're talking about now is highly relevant to this change in worldview, and the fact that none of us really know the answers is part of where we are. We're exploring, we're trying to find a new path and a new way of bringing together into coherence traditional views, modern views, scientific technical views, studies of the brain, and so forth, each in our own way.

DISCUSSION OF

Morphic Resonance, Psychedelic Experience, and Collective Memory

DAVID LUKE: Thank you very much, Rupert. I'd like to jump in first, if I may, to corroborate experientially what you were saying about psychedelics and morphic resonance. When Albert Hofmann was given *Psilocybe* mushrooms and was isolating their active alkaloids, such as psilocybin, he gave them to people who naively did not know their provenance, and they would often have visions of Aztec temples, Mayan temples, Mayan artwork, Aztec artwork, and this kind of thing. He suggested it was a kind of psychometry of the actual molecule itself, resonating with the original users.

I happen to have another observation from my own experiences working with the Huichol people of Mexico, who use peyote cactus. My first time going to their community in the Sierra, without even taking any peyote but just being there and entering into their community, every time I closed my eyes I was having visions of their cosmology—the deer, the peyote, and this kind of thing—and it was indistinguishable from when I did later take peyote; it was the same experience. It was that strong—the resonance of those people having a cosmological belief in a magical reality for such a long time.

RUPERT SHELDRAKE: Fascinating, thanks.

SANTHA FAIIA: I just want to ask, you said, "when you were an atheist." What changed?

SHELDRAKE: What stopped me being an atheist?

FAIIA: Yes.

SHELDRAKE: Well, I bought into the atheist worldview as part of my scientific education; it was a package deal. It still is for most people who study science. People who study anything at university nowadays, it turns most of them into atheists, because the assumption is we live in a totally secular world. Science has figured it all out; its dogmas of materialism are not seen as dogmas, they are seen as truths. So I just accepted that, because it's what everyone around me seemed to think, and there were two big bonuses for becoming an atheist.

First, you can have free love; I mean sex was no longer prohibited.

[Audience laughter.]

That was atheism's biggest selling point at the time. The other thing is that it gives people a sense of superiority, you know: "We now know that the world is nothing but matter," and, "People used to think that there were all these mythic beings, gods, goddesses, etcetera, but we've risen above it because we're smart, modern, educated people." There's a kind of patronizing way of looking on any religion as full of stupid deluded people who've been brainwashed by priests, and so forth, and that was just standard. I mean I see it happening the whole time today to young people. As they go to university, they emerge with this flat-tened worldview. A few break out of it, and they mainly break out of it the way I did, through taking psychedelics.

So that was one thing. For me the other thing was traveling in India in 1968 and 1969. I lived in Asia for a year—India, Sri Lanka, and I lived in Malaysia—and being in Asian cultures where perfectly sane people had completely different views of the world and didn't seem to me stu-pid and deluded, which is what I thought they would be from my athe-ist point of view, made me rethink. So then I took up Transcendental Meditation and got interested in exploring realms of the mind and yoga. I had a job in India after that and found myself unexpectedly drawn back to a Christian path, so I lived in the ashram of Father Bede Griffiths, in south India. He was my principal teacher there.

So for me it was a long journey. But I think one of the interesting things that's going on at the moment is that many people now have been brought up atheist, or agnostic, or have parents who have no interest whatsoever in religion, and they are sort of rediscovering spirituality and indeed religion. *Anatheism* is a word that means "back to God," and I think what we are seeing now is a kind of rediscovery of God in various forms—you know, Sat Chit Ananda, the spirit, shamanic paths to finding other realities—there's a huge spiritual journey going on at the moment. Mostly it's not happening through traditional organized religions, but personally I think there's a great deal to be said for organized religion. I attend church regularly, and I think it's very important to have these traditions.

FAIIA: So how would you define it? You use the term "God." You know there's this confusion as to what is God?

SHELDRAKE: What is God?

FAIIA: Yes, who is God, and how would you define him? There are all these people doing psychedelics, and this comes under the umbrella— if I understand you correctly—of the term "God"; is that what you're saying?

SHELDRAKE: Well, I'm saying that my understanding of God now is based on this idea I was talking about, Sat Chit Ananda, the nature of consciousness as the source of all things. It's more based on experience, and I think ultimately all views of God, all religious traditions, start from this experience and then are put into human languages, myths, scriptures, rituals, temples, and so on. But I think it all comes back to this direct experience, and for me that's the central part. Of course many people tell you to believe these things; that you have to take it on authority. Well, isn't that true of science, even more so? I mean how many people actually spend months in large hadron colliders figuring out the nature of quarks? Most of what we're taught about science—almost everything that most people know about science—is taken entirely on authority.

ROBIN CARHART-HARRIS: I would challenge that. It's about asking clear questions, formulating clear questions, and then testing them in a careful way. So to say that the idea that memories have storage in the brain rests on dogmatic assumption would be quite insulting to people who've done careful research into that area and have tested—with clear questions—found data, and then were able to make clear inferences based on approaching a problem with clear questions.

SHELDRAKE: Oh, I'm totally in favor of clear questions. I do experimental research all the time myself, and I try to ask clear questions. So for the question: Is memory stored in the brain? the clear questions I'd ask are, so if it's not in the brain, and if it's a resonant phenomenon, then shouldn't you be able to train an animal to learn a trick and other animals should be able to pick it up even though they're not having all those memory molecules and things? If you can get a transfer of learning, then this would suggest a transfer of memory. It's a clear question; the experiment suggests something like that is going on. I'm totally in favor of science as a way to ask clear questions.

What I'm saying is that most people who go to school and learn about science—people who graduate from university with degrees in English or drama or something like that—have not spent months or years in laboratories doing science, but they take it on authority. What I'm saying is the vast majority, most of what you learn as an undergraduate in science, you take on authority. For instance, this is the way the Krebb's cycle works, this is how DNA . . .

CARHART-HARRIS: But science is about asking questions and testing them—I think that's the critical thing. It's not belief, it's not a leap of faith; it's that something has been asked and we've looked at the data, and then we've been able to make inferences based on evidence, based on tests. It's not taking it on authority, is it?

SHELDRAKE: Well, you have a rosier view than me. For example, I do experiments and try to ask clear questions about telepathy. I'm running telephone telepathy tests at the moment. They are online, and anyone in the room can do them. They're fun, they're giving clear-cut results, and yet you know, if I appear in most scientific institutions saying, "Here I'm asking clear questions about telepathy, and here are the experiments, here's the data," then some people say, "It's great to see the evidence." But you wouldn't believe how many people—perhaps you would believe—are entirely hostile to the idea of doing the research at all, and there are organized groups of skeptics, there are militant materialists, there are people like Richard Dawkins, who are incredibly angry that anyone should be allowed to do this research. I get attacked by people who claim to be defending science based on evidence, asking clear questions, etcetera. Some people in science are sincere and do it, I think, correctly, but it has become an ideology for a lot of people, a worldview.

CARHART-HARRIS: I don't see that. I mean the idea that science is a religion that rests on some kind of leap of faith, I just don't think it holds up, because the scientific method is one of testing. It's one that, to your credit, you practice yourself. The idea of these scientists who are so narrow-minded that they won't allow you to test something like telepathy is problematic. They should allow that.

SHELDRAKE: Yes, of course they should.

GRAHAM HANCOCK: Can I add something to that? Rupert and I both had talks that we did at TEDx on the same day that were both banned by TED.* Fundamentally, the reason they banned them is that they have a scientific board that said the notion of nonlocal consciousness is pseudoscience, and therefore it must not be considered. This is ideology, this is dogma; this is not science. It's a reference frame that is being taken as a fact that isn't a fact, and it's not proven, and the research has not been done.

---

*TED is an online lecture hosting site, and TEDx is a franchise of online lectures organized independently but hosted under the TED umbrella.

CARHART-HARRIS: I think that's wrong. I think people should hear these ideas and then be able to assess the evidence that supports them.

SHELDRAKE: Well, I agree. In my recent book *The Science Delusion,* I take the ten fundamental dogmas of science and show how we could actually look at these dogmas and treat them as hypotheses that we test instead of saying they *must* be true. So my entire approach is to do science by using scientific methods.

CARHART-HARRIS: The motivation for me to say something was feeling that sometimes the scientific perspective was talked about—in an environment like this—in a slightly derogatory way, so I just wanted to address that for the sake of balance . . .

SHELDRAKE: Oh yes, I think that's fine, I'm not being derogatory. I mean I spend my entire time doing scientific experiments. I'm pro science; it's what I do. I'm anti scientific dogma, and I encounter quite a lot of it, but I'm pro science as an experimental method, and looking at evidence and hypotheses—I'm totally pro that.

WILL ROWLANDSON: Rupert, I'll start with a little anecdote, because I feel that there's a tension present in so many locations. Again it's reflected in what you've just been discussing with Robin; there's a tension between what we're taught as being explanatory models of reality and what our experience suggests. I was, I don't know, seven or eight years old, and there was a big old house near where I lived that was being rebuilt; it was all gutted. It was a sunny day, and my father decided to stop the car, and we walked into the building. It was a sunny midday, and we walked in, my mother, my father, and I, and within two seconds my mother and I ran out. We got back in the car, and we were really, *really* alarmed. My father walked in and talked to the builders; he was fine. He came out saying, "What happened to you?" And my mother and I never managed to explain it except for the fact that we both picked up something horrendous in that building. We couldn't articulate what it was.

Now it was only later when I was reading Arthur C. Clarke books—and I had loads of them as a kid—that I came across Lethbridge and his research into his theories that ghosts are memories in locations, and in particular he had the idea that they were generally around water. He had some kind of idea that water was related, but I don't know how far he pursued that. And what I was realizing is that Arthur C. Clarke was compiling theories that are held to be, as Graham [Hancock] just said, pseudo theories. These are people who are looking at fringe areas—you know, bigfoot, and foofighters, and what not. You know, "This is all the paranormal, this is all the nonnormal," and I realized my entire life was completely full of nonnormal events. So there's that tension, which I think is a tension that we're talking about in all the discussions here, between the fact that we are all talking about experiences that we have all had, and continue to, set against a model that does not accommodate them! And nonlocalized consciousness is a good example of that.

SHELDRAKE: I agree, I think that is a big problem. We have an official worldview that doesn't even accommodate consciousness in it, so the problem is that it's a kind of denial. For example, I did my research on dogs that know when their owners are coming home. I did this because thousands of people told me they had dogs that knew when they were coming home, so I decided to investigate it—do experiments, film the dog, have people come at random times, and so forth. The results were successful, and positive, and I've since been trying to persuade people to do this research in universities. There have been plenty of students who wanted to take it up, but their supervisors have invariably said to them, "You know, I'm personally sympathetic, and I think it's a really interesting question, but if you want to be a scientist you'll kill your career right from the outset if you do research on telepathy."

And they're right. And so things that are very much part of daily experience—other things I've looked at such as telephone telepathy and the sense of being stared at—are things that, despite being part of daily or frequent experience, are completely banned from this world-view. If people try to do research on them at universities, they're usually stopped, because it doesn't fit the paradigm. I think that what we need to do is find a model of reality that includes all that's good about science but without the dogmatic exclusions that exclude so much of experience. I think the job of science is to investigate what happens, so I actually try to investigate these things scientifically. I think that's how we should do it and that science would benefit from being wider and more inclusive.

JEREMY NARBY: Well, Rupert, it's always a pleasure to listen to you. As I was preparing for my talk yesterday, I looked into the etymology of the word *spirit,* and this led me back to the Bible and the breath of God. So I was reading the Bible as an agnostic a couple of weeks ago and googling "the breath of God," and it seems that it's a little less clear-cut than the idea that God insufflated his breath only into humans; there are other passages that indicate that he insufflated his breath into all living creatures.

SHELDRAKE: Yes.

NARBY: Nevertheless the idea that humans are in his image has been a strong idea and has marked a lot of Western Judeo-Christian culture, so there seem to be several strains within Christian theology on that. What is your view on that question?

SHELDRAKE: Well, I think the word *spirit* means breath, or wind, and has a whole variety of meanings, and in the Jewish Bible—the Old Testament—it's a bit makeshift—there's little bits here and there, but it's not a systematic exposition of theory. For a systematic and coherent attempt to put this into a kind of philosophical frame-work, you really have to look at the church fathers and Origen, whom Peter [Meyer] referred to yesterday, from the third and fourth century; they're mainly Neoplatonic, but they were influenced by Greek philosophy.

The challenge of the early Christian philosophers was to bring together these rather crude Jewish metaphors, very concrete metaphors, with all the sophistication of classical philosophy. The New Testament was written in Greek, so these worlds collided, and what came out of it was a synthesis; the doctrine of the Holy Trinity, which is the principal conception of God that they arrived at in the first few centuries, includes the spirit as part of the divine nature—the spirit being the principle of energy, movement, and change in the whole of nature.

Now the spirit is also that which inspires and can inspire human beings, and human beings reflect God through having minds that reflect the divine mind. But according to Saint Bonaventure and the Franciscan school, those in the Western church extended this very explicitly to the whole of nature, to plants and animals as well. In the Greek Orthodox tradition, the spirit was much more central to the whole of their theology; the spirit of God is the breath of life in all nature and is the energy in all nature—that's pretty mainstream in Greek theology. So the Bible itself has undeveloped hints that were later put together into a more coherent system.

But of course there are different schools: Greek orthodox, Russian orthodox, Anglican, Catholic; there are many different types of theology. But if you go back to the formative theologies and the doctrine of the Holy Trinity—which was their best attempt to understand the nature of God as not just being an undifferentiated being and certainly not an old man with a beard but as having different attributes that are recognizable—then being is one of them. The "ground of all being" [that God is the basis of all being, as Paul Tillich holds] is fundamental, and consciousness or knowledge is another aspect of God. But that in itself would lead to a kind of static Platonic realm, and you wouldn't get a world full of movement and change. So then there has to be this dynamical principle. They're not separate, they're all united together.

Then theologians and mystics like Meister Eckhart in the Middle Ages said all these are just conceptions. How can our limited minds ever conceive of God? And that the true God, the godhead, is behind all these models. In Greek theology their official school of theology is *apophatic,* which means, "We can only say what God is not; we can say these are ways of understanding God that our minds can grasp, but they point to a reality that is by its very nature far greater than anything we can conceive." The best we can do is experience it through direct intuition or mystical experience. So I would say those were the mainstream positions. You then get the Protestant Reformation people who say, "Oh no, forget all this tradition, forget what these people have said, and we'll just read the Bible. It's literally true." That's a kind of modern deviation. American fundamentalism, which was invented in the early twentieth century and has almost no relation to this traditional theology, rejects, or actually it's just ignorant of, this entire school of thought.

ROWLANDSON: Just ignorant!

[Audience laughter.]

BERNARD CARR: Rupert, I'd like to start off going back to the first point you made about this transformation in the nature of science because I think it's really important. Just last year there was this postmaterialist manifesto where a large number, maybe a hundred, scientists signed this, basically saying that we have to expand our concept of science to accommodate the sort of phenomena we're talking about and that really the distinction is between science and scientism. To address what Robin [Carhart-Harris] said, no one is denying the importance of science, but it's this scientism, which is a sort of fundamentalist form of science that says that the material world is all there is, consciousness is produced by the brain, and that's it. That's what is really being argued. Scientism is in relation to science, in some sense, as fundamentalist religions are to more enlightened spirituality. I think one hundred is a small number and doesn't represent the majority view of scientists, but it's a growing movement I think, and well, Christianity started with twelve people, so it seems to me it's a small movement, but I think it is a growing one. It's sort of a trend.

Science has to expand. There's nothing wrong with the scientific method; the problem is the idea that there's this one form of reality, this material world, and that's the only form of reality. I think what one learns from all of these mystical experiences people are talking about is that there are other levels of reality. Somehow that has to be accommodated within a more enlightened scientific worldview. I personally like the view of the primacy of consciousness, the sort of Hindu view that there are different levels of consciousness—you know, planetary, galactic—and that one can access different intelligences; we've heard a lot about that in this meeting.

But what intrigues me now is the question, What is the relationship among all these different types of consciousness? I mean, for example, we've heard how through DMT you can access Andrew [Gallimore]'s mechanical beings and how through ayahuasca you can detect the plant beings and then through mystical experience you have other levels of experience, such as interacting with other levels of consciousness, of intelligence; but my question is if there is this entire hierarchy of consciousness with which one can interact, then how does it all fit together? I mean, for example, in drug experiences can I, in principle, experience the full-blown mystical state you can get by going to a cave for fifteen years and meditating? Are there different domains that one can access through drug experiences or is everything open to it?

SHELDRAKE: Well, I think this is a question for research and consciousness studies. I mean, there were people who used to say psychedelic experience is a kind of cheat and real mystical experience is something quite different. I don't believe that; I think that they're very closely related. And people can access different states through meditation. There's all sorts of altered states of consciousness: you can arrive at them through meditation; you can arrive at them through experiences in nature such as mystical connection with nature; you can arrive at them through drugs; you can arrive at them through near-death experiences. And there are many ways to alter our consciousness and contact other realms—through rituals, liturgy, and chanting to name a few.

So conducting the cartography of these different realms of consciousness can only be done through conscious exploration. You know this is happening now; it's happened always. I mean the great Rishis in India, the great seers in their caves, were doing this, and the monks in the Egyptian desert, the early Christian monks, who were spending years and years meditating and finding out about their minds from within. Lots of people have done it over the centuries in all sorts of different ways and in all sorts of different traditions. And as you know, if you look at the *Journal of Consciousness Studies* now, you can find papers there on ayahuasca experiences, meditation, and altered states of consciousness of different kinds. So this is actually now happening as an exploration, and I don't think we know the answers as to how similar or how different these states are.

EDE FRECSKA: Is the morphogenetic field within our space-time or outside of it, and how do its effects spread if it is within our space-time?

SHELDRAKE: Well, it's in. My morphogenetic field's within and around me, so it's like a magnetic field. It's localized around and within the system it organizes. So they're localized fields, but morphic resonance is nonlocal in the sense that what happens here now, for instance, if I learn something now, then this can have an effect on someone somewhere else. How does that influence spread? As I've said, I don't know.

There have been various people who have tried to explain this in terms of variations of quantum theory. David Bohm was very interested in morphic resonance, and as you know, he was a leading quantum physicist. He and I had a long discussion about it, and he had this idea that underlying the world we live in—the phenomenal world—is what he called the implicate order. The implicate order unfolds into the explicate order, or the phenomenal world. But the implicate order is not itself in space and time, or at least it's in other dimensions of space and time. It's not in three- or four-dimensional space and time. So as I said to Bohm, if you just have the implicate order giving the explicate order, then you've just reinvented Neoplatonism—you've got a kind of platonic realm that folds out to the phenomenal world.

But we live in an evolutionary universe, and if the explicate order can modify the implicate order, then it would have a memory, and Bohm adopted this as part of his theory. So you've got the idea that things that happen can influence the implicate order by giving it a kind of memory. The implicate order then has this accumulative memory and can act anywhere at any time. If a rat learns a new trick in London, then it changes the implicate order, so when rats learn a similar trick or the same trick somewhere else, they learn it quicker. So through modifying his theory of quantum physics, he arrived at the same predictions as I make on the basis of morphic resonance. Now, Bernard [Carr] has a multidimensional theory of physics that might also be another way of mapping this onto a physical model. And there are probably other ways of doing it . . .

LUIS LUNA: Who is the theorist?

SHELDRAKE: Bernard Carr.

LUKE: He's sat behind you.

LUNA: Oh, okay!

[Audience laughter. Luis turns around, and Bernard waves hello.]

SHELDRAKE: Bernard Carr is a cosmologist, but he's been interested in psychical research and consciousness research for many years and has taken his own adaptation of what's now mainstream in physics: multidimensional reality, superstring theory, and M-theory, which are all multidimensional. In the 1920s occasionally people said, "Well, maybe the mind and things like telepathy involve an extra dimension," and everyone got terribly upset at the idea of an extra dimension. Extra dimensions come cheap nowadays; physics is full of them!

[Audience laughter.]

FRECSKA: I am asking if quantum is involved: Is it possible that future habits morph present habits?

SHELDRAKE: You mean an influence from the future?

FRECSKA: Basically, yes, some future influence. I'm thinking how to avoid Neoplatonism.

SHELDRAKE: Oh, well, I avoid Neoplatonism because Neoplatonism doesn't have a memory, you see, and I think that the problem with classical Western philosophy and the problem with science—because it's so based on Greek philosophy—is that it's not evolutionary. The Platonic world of ideas, or the Pythagorean world of mathematical forms, is an eternal world beyond space and time that doesn't evolve. In the eighteenth and nineteenth century most physicists thought the universe was made up of eternal matter and energy and governed by eternal laws.

Since 1966, we've had an evolutionary cosmology. The whole universe evolves, starting less than the size of the head of a pin and billions of degrees centigrade, and it's been growing ever since. But they still think all the laws of nature were completely fixed at the moment of the Big Bang. That's a hangover from the Platonic cosmology. When I suggest that these may not be fixed laws but are in fact habits, then this comes up against a dogma, and they say, "No, you can't say that because the laws of nature are fixed." "Why?" "Well, because they are."

And then they get into terrible problems: "Why are they fixed just right for us to exist in this universe?" Then either they say there has to be an intelligent designer, a neodeistic view, or you have to have a multiverse, which is trillions of universes, to explain how we're in this one; we just happen to be in the one that's right for us, but all the others actually exist. Bernard Carr is at the center of this; he's edited the main book called *Universe or Multiverse?* He knows much more about this debate than I do.

I think if you drop the idea that all the laws are fixed, a lot of this discussion goes away, because if the habits of nature can evolve, then they don't all have to be fixed right at the beginning, and you don't have the question of why are they as they are at the beginning. But I think the Platonic universe is one that doesn't evolve. We live in a universe that does evolve, and Western thought, the basis of our thinking, has an evolutionary part. The Judeo-Christian part of our history is all about developmental processes in time. The prototypic journey is when the people of Israel get out of Egypt through the wilderness to the promised land. The primary metaphor is a journey, and history is a journey. The secularized version of that is progress, and we've converted the whole world to it, but it comes out of Judeo-Christian roots.

The idea of timeless order comes from Greek roots, and that has had a stronger influence on physics. That's why I think we have this particular problem, and why any evolutionary theory with the idea of habits and memory allows us to have forms that are not Platonic forms because they're evolving forms, and they can evolve along with the cosmos. That's why I think we need an evolutionary conception of natural order as opposed to a fixed Platonic one.

ERIK DAVIS: This is a sharper and more theological version of Bernard [Carr]'s question about entities and hierarchy, and it takes the form of the following: It seems to me that one of the significant differences between Christian neo-orthodox theology and, let's say, a Hindu model is that in the Hindu model you do not really have anything that is equivalent to a Satanic principle. Both through the mechanism of reincarnation as a cycle of moving through karma and through the emphasis on nondualism, you avoid the problem of evil in a certain way. Without getting into the intricacies, I'm interested in particular when you talk about reading psychedelics from a perspective of a divine mind, how do you respond? And what do we do more generally with the fact that there are hellish experiences and that there are demonic dimensions that people tune in to? I think you were not here the first day; did you see Graham's talk?

SHELDRAKE: Yes.

DAVIS: So there's this whole pop-culture, Lovecraftian horror show that's in popular psychedelic culture that people enjoy and are tuning in to as part, sometimes, of a spiritual path where they can confront and move through the demons, sometimes in more sort of a "Wow, that's weird man!" kind of lowbrow, pop-culture way. But I'm just curious, from your perspective, seeing this enchanted universe from a theological point of view, from your Christian point of view, how do you deal with them; how do you see those energies?

SHELDRAKE: Oh, gosh, just a little question at the end of the morning!

[Audience laughter.]

Well, nightmares are dreams in which entities are usually chasing or trying to devour us. A study of nightmares of children in New York City showed that the principal nightmares are the children feeling they're being pursued and are going to be devoured by monsters or animals. They're not about realistic dangers like being run over by cars, even though no New York child is likely to encounter a predatory wild animal.

I think that part of the stuff of nightmares comes from our long past of being animals that were prey animals for large predators. So the thing about a lot of horror films is there's these vampires, these monsters, that are going to get you, eat you, and devour you. So I think part of that element is not so much evil as a kind of morphic-resonance memory of realistic dreams of being eaten by tigers. At the beginning of the twentieth century, every year thousands of people were killed by tigers in India. This is not something that far away. I think part of it is that; I don't think that's evil. I think the idea of people who are utterly evil, the idea that there are these totally evil forces, is an ambiguity in most traditions.

Certainly in the Christian tradition there's an ambiguity about whether evil is an autonomous force, and if so then how does it originate; or as Aquinas thought of it, is evil a privation of the good? For example, Aquinas's discussion of the fall of angels is very interesting: in the hierarchy of angels there are nine levels; the top level is seraphim, cherubim, and thrones—like cosmic archetypes. The seraphim are the angels of divine love, the thrones are the angels of divine presence, and the cherubim are the angels of divine knowledge. It's only the cherubim that could fall. An angel that is in the presence of the divine couldn't fall from grace because it's constantly in divine presence. An angel that's burning with divine love can't fall because it's all about love, but the angel of knowledge can fall because knowledge can be perverted and become a source of pride.

So the fall of Satan is not because knowledge is bad, but because of the desire to become autonomous and no longer be part of the cosmic order. So the idea in Aquinas that I find the most satisfactory, really, is that evil people are not evil usually because they want to be evil, but because they think they are doing good. I mean Hitler thought he was doing good for the Germans, for example. He didn't say, "I'm going to wreck my country, and I hate Germany"—no, but he had a limited conception of whom he should do good for.

What about sexual predators? Sex itself is not bad, and the drive toward orgasm and pleasure is part of our animal nature. But if to satisfy that involves killing people because it makes the predators more thrilled to kill people in the process of having sex with them, then that becomes evil because it's a form of predation, where their naturally good desires become a limited good where they're no longer about anyone else's good, just their own.

I find that a more plausible way. I think the kind of gothic horror side of these evil forces perhaps exists, but I think they're more a problem of imagination and fantasy than of anything else. Of course, psychedelic states lend themselves to the creation of fantastical imagery, and if one went into a psychedelic state expecting to see monsters, and if one had a solid diet of horror films, I imagine that nightmarish scenarios would become quite common. Luckily I've never had that kind myself. I have had nightmarish experiences, bad trips, sometimes, but they haven't dominated the whole thing, and usually I pray before I go into these experiences, and I pray during them too, for guidance and help, and I find that really works.

LUKE: I'd like to draw it to a close there and thank Rupert for a wonderful presentation.

CHAPTER 9

Psychedelics, Entities, Dark Matter, and Parallel Dimensions

Graham Hancock

I know it's boring to hear other people's trip reports—but can I begin with a short trip report?

This happened on a friend's ranch. I have had lots of amazing DMT experiences, wonderful, lovely, healing experiences, so when I went back there—just prior to flying down to Brazil to Luis Eduardo Luna's retreat at Wasiwaska—I was expecting that my DMT experience would be the same loving, healing, beautiful experience that I'd had before. But it wasn't, and I just want to read this to you:

> When I found myself back at the same location I felt relaxed and welcomed what I expected would be another pleasant healing excursion to the DMT realms. I certainly had no expectation that anything particularly disturbing or terrifying would happen to me. Turned out I was wrong.
>
> As soon as I took my first long draw I had the unsettling feeling that something intelligent and not necessarily friendly had leapt

into my head from the spherical glass pipe. I held in the smoke as long as I could, then took another long draw. By now there was a crackling, buzzing sound in my ears, and I felt utterly overwhelmed and had to lie back at once. I always lie back, no way can I stay sitting up! Immediately things were very different, though with some similarities from all my previous smoked DMT experiences.

The first thing I saw was something like a mandala with an ivory background and intricate brick-red geometric lines—like tracks—inside it. Between the lines, or tracks, imposed on the ivory background were a large number of clock faces with weird hands. I've seen something like this before, not under smoked DMT, but under a very strong dose of ayahuasca. It terrified me then, don't know why, and it proceeded to terrify me again. Then I realized that the mandala—only an approximation, there was something very like computer circuitry about it as well, or even like one of those toy race car tracks where little electric cars whizz round and round—was sentient and focused on me.

I got a hint of eyes or feelers. There was something very menacing about the whole scene, and I began to feel uncomfortable and restless in my body and had enough of my everyday consciousness left at that point to wish profoundly that I hadn't smoked the pipe, and felt myself struggling—uselessly of course—against the effect. Then I heard an ominous voice, filled with a sort of malicious glee, that said very clearly, "YOU'RE OURS NOW." And I thought, shit, yes, I am yours now, not much I can do about it, but it's only for about ten more minutes and then I'm out of here.

Since it was pointless to struggle, I resigned myself to the situation and thought, okay then, get on with it, and immediately the mandala/intelligence and lots of its little helpers (whom I felt but cannot describe) were all over me. I had the sense that my body was a huge, fat, bloated cocoon and that these beings were tearing it apart, tearing off lumps of matter and throwing them aside, getting access to the real, hidden me. I was aware that this was a place of absolute truth, like the Hall of Maat in the ancient Egyptian tradition, and that everything about me was known here, every thought, every action, good and bad, throughout the whole of my life—and the sense that the real hidden me within the cocoon was utterly transparent to these beings and that they were finding me wanting. About as far from being "justified in the judgment"—as the Egyptian texts put it—as it is possible to be and that therefore I might face annihilation here.

And I heard something like a trumpet blast and a loud voice that announced, as though this were a proclamation at court: "NOW THE GREAT UNFOLDING WILL BEGIN." Or possibly: "NOW THE GREAT TRANSFORMATION WILL BEGIN."

This was the point where I lost consciousness of the material realm completely, and indeed of everything else. Feeling utterly helpless, utterly in the power of whatever process I was going through and of the intelligence that was running it, I fell into a darkness that seemed to last forever. I have no conscious recollection of what happened to me in there, only the conviction that it was something massive. When I began to come out of it there were some moments—though this felt much longer than moments—when I was deeply confused and disoriented and had absolutely no idea where I was or why I was there.

I could see the room around me but didn't recognize it, didn't even know it was a room at first, or even what a room is, and it kept melting back into that other terrifying reality out of which I was emerging. This has never happened to me with DMT before—I've always known, even in the depths of the experience, that I was having that experience because I had smoked a pipe of DMT and my body was in a specific place, which I did not forget, at a specific time. This was completely different and very, very scary.

Gradually my eyes began to focus. I remembered I had smoked DMT. I looked around and saw Santha [Faiia] sitting on the edge of the bed, very calm and incredibly strong. I was immersed in a wild melting storm of colors and the only clear sure thing in the whole place for me was Santha, with her amazing strength and beauty, and lines of light emerging from her body and rising up out of her and surrounding her. I remember falling to my knees on the floor in front of her and telling her, "I found you again" or something such. I had the sense that I had known her in a past life and had found her again in this one. And I also told her that she is a goddess. I felt shaken, but basically happy to be back on planet normal. I was able to witness the sessions of several other participants without actually falling apart or melting down.

After that, Santha and I flew to Brazil, and there I had five sessions of ayahuasca with Luis Eduardo [Luna]. During those five sessions of ayahuasca I had experiences that were extremely powerful. The net effect was that it stopped me using cannabis completely for three years. I'd been using it all day long for decades, but suddenly I just stopped completely; so there was a transformation of a kind. I am using cannabis again now, in small quantities in the form of an oil, but it definitely intervened and changed an aspect of my life.

This presentation will broadly cover the material I explored in *Supernatural* and which I and others have explored in our new book *The Divine Spark*.

Altered states of consciousness, or trance states, are the universal feature that's common to all shamanism, whether in the remote past or today. In these altered states of consciousness, it's very common for shamans to report encounters with intelligent supernatural entities, which they usually construe as spirits. The spirits that shamans encounter can sometimes take human form, can sometimes appear as an animal-human hybrid known as a therianthrope or they can take the form of spirit animals. Shamans of all cultures report that they themselves transform into animals, or therianthropes, during their trance journeys in the spirit world.

Many of the experiences that shamans report with spirits are very similar—at the phenomenological level—with encounters with aliens reported by tens of thousands of people in the West who believe they've been abducted by UFOs, and yet supposedly the domains of spirits and aliens are completely separate. In ayahuasca paintings these days, shamans themselves very frequently depict UFOs and aliens, giving a sense of a connection with a wider and more mysterious cosmos. Such is the case with examples from Pablo Amaringo: a flying saucer there, alien-like beings, and there a human-headed serpent.

If we want a database on the phenomenology of shamanism, Mircea Eliade is as good a place to start as any, and if we want a database on the phenomenology of UFO abduction experiences, the late John Mack left us with a fabulous body of work, a huge dossier of experiences, that can be drawn on. And others, like Budd Hopkins and David Jacobs, have contributed to that dossier of UFO abductees.

These two apparently very different domains turn out to have a lot in common. The spirits that shamans most frequently encounter first appear as animals, birds, fish, or therianthropes. John Mack summed that up: "The aliens appear to be consummate shape shifters, often appearing initially to abductees as animals: owls, eagles, racoons, and deer are among the creatures the abductees have seen initially." And here are some examples from Virginia Horton, a UFO abductee. She's talked with an intelligent grey deer that she feels has a person inside it. Another abductee reports seeing a deer through her window just before she was abducted. Another sees a wolf standing squarely on her bed.

Shamans routinely report being floated up into the sky, or climbing up on a rope of light, or being drawn up in a thread of light, and in the San rock art of South Africa you can see those themes manifested. A Bushman shaman from Botswana says, "I dance, when I emerge I am already climbing, I climb the threads, I take them and climb them, then I follow the thread to the wells, the ones I am going to enter, the thread to the wells of metal. When you get to the wells you duck beneath the pieces of metal."

These experiences, whether they be climbing a thread of light or being taken up to an object in the sky, seem to be essentially the same in the UFO abductee realm and in the shamanic and spirit realm, at the level of phenomenology.

Shamans are frequently abducted to the sky, but they are also abducted underwater or into caves, and again that turns out to be the case with UFO abductees. Betty Aho describes being plunged into the sea, into huge crystalline caverns; Filiberto Cardenas is taken to a beach and taken to a tunnel beneath the sea; Carlos Diaz sees, eventually, a UFO in a cave. The parallels with shamanistic phenomenology are quite intriguing, and the most obvious one is the shamanic ordeal—the tortures and piercings that are inflicted on shamans by spirits as part of their initiation, including the insertion of objects into their bodies.

All kinds of accounts from all over the world tell of bizarre surgical procedures in the hands of spirits who implant various objects into people. This is absolutely the most common, widely known aspect of the UFO abduction experiences, which is that the abductee experiences surgery at the hands of the aliens. There are curious parallels between these domains. Sandra Larson, a UFO abductee, tells us that beings removed her brain and set it down beside her; while a Yakut shaman speaks of the spirits—the spirits cut off his head and set it aside. Bone-counting experiences occur in both domains; it's again very similar phenomenology.

Shamans, of course, often report having sex with spirits and frequently have hybrid offspring in the spirit realm, and that again is identical at a phenomenological level with the UFO abductee experience because UFO abductees are frequently having sex with aliens, have lovers in the alien realm, and have hybrid children there. In Alex Grey's painting from the front of Rick Strassman's wonderful book *The Spirit Molecule*, we can see that eyes are a constant theme of the DMT experience. And curiously, in the twelfth century *Rupertsberg Codex*, we see eyes in the sky, even in a similar diamond shape to the drawing from the Cash-Landrum UFO sighting in the 1960s. Further, in the *Rupertsberg* image, there's this curious umbilical coming down from the diamond-shaped object in the sky—it must be in the sky because there are stars—that turns out to be connected to a fetus in the womb of a woman; and then oddly enough there's a little elf, or imp, in the picture, and what is he holding but a mushroom. I wonder what that mushroom contained.

If we look at a 1710 painting of the baptism of Christ, what the hell is going on here? There's a flying saucer in a painting from 1710! It's really bizarre. You can see mysterious books, a sense of mission, and healing powers in the image. Shamans are often, it turns out, if you read the literature, given books by spirits. Maria Sabina was given a book. She said she learned many things from it—"it helped people who need help and to know the secrets of the world where everything is known"—but she wasn't allowed to keep the book; it remained in the sky. Same thing happened to Betty Hill. She was given a large book by the aliens, but they reclaimed it before she left the ship. Betty Andreasson was given a small blue book with forty luminous pages, but it soon afterward disappeared. Both shamans and UFO abductees tend to have a sense of mission, of being entrusted with deep knowledge, and with healing powers that they need to share with the rest of the human race at some point.

What about fairies and elves, and why do they have so much in common with aliens and spirits? Of course, the go-to book on this subject is Jacques Vallee's *Passport to Magonia,* which is, I think, the first book that really explored the phenomenological similarity between fairies and aliens. That book was published in 1969. A lot has happened in these realms since then, and in my book *Supernatural* I updated that dossier of comparing these supposedly different realms. Fairies, just like spirits, just like aliens, were in the business of abducting people. They were renowned and feared for that. There are eerie accounts of people seeing fairies dancing in a ring that they feel compelled to approach, but if they touch that ring of dancing fairies, they'll be suddenly transported to another world.

There are frequent reports of individuals who feel they have spent three or four hours in fairyland, but when they come back, three or four hundred years have passed and they've returned to an utterly transformed world. That's a bit like the missing-time phenomenon in UFO abductions, except in that case it's usually only three or four hours in this realm that have been lost, not three or four centuries. It's almost as if the technology has gotten better.

This whirling circular nature of the fairy dance reminds me a little bit of flying saucers, actually. Maybe there are other realms, and evolution is taking place in those, and maybe the technology for crossing dimensional space has changed; it was a dance, now it's a flying saucer.

Fairies could be cruel; they tortured and hurt human beings. They could be kind; they gave gifts to people and healing powers—again the parallels with spirits and aliens. Fairies had the power of flight—they made use of aerial vehicles, flying boats, flying castles, flying carriages, etcetera—and fairies often also abduct people underground, into the hollow caves beneath the earth. In one classic fairy picture you can see a door in the side of the hollow hills, fairies dancing in a circle, and what looks suspiciously like *Amanita muscaria* in the foreground.

In another image a young man is being seduced by a group of fairy maids who are seeking to entice him into fairyland, and again there's something fungal down there on the ground. Fairies and elves often appear in the form of animals or part-animal, part-human hybrids. In a fifteenth-century woodcut from Holland, we can see a group of fairies dancing in a circle; they are classic therianthropes, part-animal, part-human in form.

A medieval fairy was feared because she abducted human babies, and she would often take the form of a part-serpent, part-human hybrid. In seventeenth-century Scotland, there are many reports of women being abducted to nurse fairy babes and describing the place they are taken to, and this is extremely similar to the re-abduction of UFO abductees who have a hybrid offspring in the alien realm and are constantly re-abducted to nurture and care for that offspring.

Basically, my sense is that, as human beings, we cannot perceive something without interpreting it. Interpretation is built into perception from the get-go, and our perceptions are structured by the culture and the society in which we live. What I'm suggesting is that these three supposedly different domains of fairies, spirits, and aliens are actually the same very ancient and long-lived phenomenon of human experience viewed through different cultural spectacles and experienced by different people in different periods of history. So how far can we trace this phenomenon back?

As a reminder of some of the common forms in which aliens, spirits, and fairies all appear, if we look at the oldest surviving cave art in the world—well, it's actually been surpassed recently by a piece from Indonesia, but the art from Fumane Cave in Italy is thirty-five thousand years old—we see a human body with the head and horns of some kind of auroch, probably, or some kind of ancestor of cattle. And in the Hohlenstein-Stadel Cave in Germany, we have a lion man, thirty-two thousand years old, carved from mammoth ivory. And in the Chauvet Cave, we have the bison man who is replicated again and again. These bison-man figures continue to appear in the painted caves for ten thousand years or more.

Sometimes we see bizarre hybrids, such as a combination of a stag, an owl, a wolf, or a horse and a human being, such as the one called "The Sorcerer." It's in the Trois Frères cave in France, and it's seventeen thousand years old. These appear to be the earliest expressions of such ideas in human culture, so we have to ask ourselves, where do they come from? What was the source, what was their inspiration? If we pull back from that Chauvet image we'll see that bison man is actually straddling a female form with a prominent pubic triangle. Yet this female form is weirdly headless, and her right arm is transforming into the head of a lion. This is clearly not something that you see out on the plains while hunting game; you don't see people transforming into bison or lions. What we are witnessing here, therefore, is a moment of transformation, shape-shifting, and I would suggest such experiences only occur in deeply altered states of consciousness.

Another example is a piece from the Pech Merle cave in France, which I've had the privilege of spending quite a bit of time in front of, and it's really quite intriguing. There's something going on in the sky here for a start, above the figure. The figure has multiple piercings. It's human in form, but look at that head, those large dark eyes. I don't think it's a big leap to say it looks a lot like our ideas of alien greys today, but it's there in a painted cave more than twenty-four thousand years ago.

There are others, from Altamira, in Spain, and Bernifal in France, and archaeologists really just don't know what they are. They're patterns, but they look a lot like the flying saucers that Pablo Amaringo painted from his ayahuasca visions in the 1980s. You can compare these ancient finger traces done on clay, more than fifteen thousand years ago, with an image drawn by one of John Mack's patients, a UFO abductee who told Mack that this image was projected into her visual field every time she was about to be abducted. I would suggest the same inspiration lies behind both images, though widely separated in time.

Let's explore the relationship of DMT and psilocybin, though I think the problem with the UFO abductee lobby is that they take an extremely nuts-and-bolts approach to this connection. I have found that people who are passionate advocates of alien contact and UFO abductions tend to be more extremely materialist even than Richard Dawkins; they want an exclusively materialistic interpretation. Obviously to them, these are physical beings like us who have high technology like us and are crossing interstellar space in spaceships. And to suggest that it might have anything to do with consciousness actually results in explosions of fury from members of that lobby—which remind me a lot of the explosions of fury of the materialist faction within science.

There is cave art trumpeted as the earliest evidence for magic mushroom use in Europe, thought to be *Psilocybe hispanica,* in a painted cave, but in fact the evidence for the deployment and harnessing of deeply altered states of consciousness goes much further back than that. There are certain distinctive features of the cave art of Europe that leave little room for doubt that psilocybin or perhaps other hallucinogens were involved from the very beginning, such as the wildly elaborated antlers from Lascaux. There's often geometrical patterns in the imagery, and elsewhere a grid between two ibexes, more grids from Altamira, and more of the same kind of thing from el Castillo in Spain. Essentially, the work that has made the breakthrough in this field is the work of Professor David Lewis-Williams at the University of Witwatersrand in South Africa.

I want to recognize Terence McKenna and his amazing insights with *Food of the Gods,* but it's important to be clear that very good academic work has been done, certainly on the role of altered states of consciousness and the development of the modern human mind, going back to the 1970s, and that's David Lewis-Williams's work. He broke a deadlock in the study of cave art with the proposal that all this art can be explained if we understand that it was an art of visions, that shamans were entering altered states of consciousness, and then, returning to the daily state of consciousness, they would remember their visions and paint them on cave walls.

The presence of therianthropes in the art and of what are called entoptic phenomena are indicative of this; these kinds of patterns are the entoptics. David Lewis-Williams partly drew on the research done with hallucinogens just before the war on drugs kicked in and stopped these intriguing areas of inquiry. In fact, the volunteers so regularly reported seeing the same patterns that it was possible to draw up a chart of these so-called entoptic phenomena and what they look like.

It's interesting to look and compare the hallucinogenic entoptic phenomena of modern volunteers with rock art of the San of southern Africa. The Kalahari Bushmen are still around, but the San are gone. There was a time in South Africa when you could actually buy a licence to hunt the San as vermin for fifty British pounds. We know, however, from ethnologists who spoke with the San at the end of the nineteenth century—those few survivors—that they did enter deeply altered states of consciousness. Not with plants, but with a trance dance around the fire.

They would sense their spirits leaving their bodies, and they would depict what they saw in their visions. Again, the same patterns occur also with the Koso in the California Great Basin. We can't send ethnographers back to talk to the Upper Paleolithic cave artists, but the patterns that they depict are the same as the patterns that we know are connected with experiences of altered states of consciousness, so it's pretty obvious that prehistoric shamans were at work. David Lewis-Williams presents this chart of supposedly different stages of the visionary experience, the entoptics, and then the sense of passing through a vortex into a seamlessly convincing parallel world. Several of the volunteers in the experiments he records depicted entities, such as the example he uses of a man in a modern business suit with the head of a fox. This was from an experiment in the '60s, and that's just the same, in concept, as the lion man or the bison man from the painted caves.

Once we accept that altered states of consciousness were involved in all the strange visionary aspects—and indeed the universal aspects—of cave art, the transcultural aspects of cave art begin to fit into place. We can understand the inspiration for such imagery; we can even experience it ourselves. We're going to be hearing from Rick [Strassman] next, but it's impossible for me to speak about this without mentioning his incredibly important work with DMT.

I am struck by the phenomenology of Rick's volunteers, and so was Rick, because a lot of the volunteers reported experiences that were pretty much like UFO-abduction experiences, except obviously they weren't being abducted because they were on a hospital bed in New Mexico. Paul sees a lot of elves, Jim has clinical researchers probing his mind, Ben feels something inserted into his left forearm, Lucas actually sees a space station with entities inside it—automatons, android-like creatures.

I of course cannot draw, but I made an image from one of my early ayahuasca experiences in the Amazon, when I encountered what I construed to be aliens and depicted one with hatched eyes like an insect. I wrote in my notes at the time: "This is not a good representation; the eyes may be bigger and are multi-segmented like those of a fly. The entity observes me dispassionately, doesn't seem good or particularly bad, then disappears. But gradually the experience became more ominous, and I became convinced that I was going to be taken, and I was filled with terror. I was sitting on a bench and I sat upright, opened my eyes, and I said out loud, 'NO!!!' and the experience stopped. And of course, what I should have done was kept my eyes closed, and said out loud, 'YES! Take me!!!' But cowardice intervened, and I have never since had that particular experience. I've had many entity encounters, but this sense of about to be taken has never come back. I made a huge mistake in saying no!"

I'm intrigued by the reports of Rick's volunteers in that a number of the volunteers met entities who seemed pleased that they had discovered the DMT technology and that it was a technology for communicating with them. Rick addresses this problem of personal inner space and shared transpersonal experiences and says that this is very challenging to the worldview of mainstream science. He recognized the similarities with UFO abduction experiences, and he proposed, cutting a long story short, that UFO abductees might be spontaneous overproducers of endogenous DMT, and that explains the experiences that they have. But that does not necessarily imply that such experiences, mediated by DMT, were in any way unreal.

I'm not aware of anything in science that allows us to reduce hallucinations to changes in the brain activity that accompany them, and the analogy I usually give is a telescope: we point it at the sky if we want to see a distant star, we focus it, physical changes take place inside the barrel of the telescope in the relationship between the lenses, and eventually the star comes into view. But we'd be completely wrong to say that the star *is* the physical changes inside the barrel of the telescope. It can't be reduced to that; those changes have simply allowed us to see it. And maybe that's what DMT is doing in the brain: it's allowing us to see something real that is not normally accessible to our senses. Like a telescope, it's a piece of technology.

Rick looks into this whole issue of the receiver model of the brain and suggests that we are normally routinely tuned in to channel normal, but DMT provides regularly repeated and reliable access to other channels. He takes the daring step of suggesting that it's just as likely that we're dealing with freestanding parallel realms as "this is all in our brains."

So maybe we have a secret doorway inside our minds, through which we can project our consciousness into other dimensions and through which intelligences in other dimensions may make contact with us and teach us stuff that we didn't know before. Maybe that's what's going on here. It's certainly intriguing that the moment our ancestors start to manifest evidence they are cultivating and deliberately inducing altered states of consciousness a kind of transformation overtakes human behavior. At that very same moment, we have stone tools, hunting tactics, and spiritual ideas all take a quantum leap forward at the same time. It's regarded as the most significant change in the whole story of the evolution of human behavior—it's just that very few scientists are connecting it to the altered state of consciousness experiences. There's definitely a correlation, and I would suggest that it's causative.

Of course, Steve Jobs and Steve Wozniak were quite honest that none of us would be holding these nice little Apple computers if it wasn't for LSD. They preferentially employed people who had had psychedelic experiences, as they felt that they would be better programmers. So here is a huge technical innovation that appears not to be attributed to the alert, problem-solving state of consciousness but to visionary experience in some way.

Now this is probably an urban legend—never believe anything you read in the *Daily Mail*—nevertheless, it's an interesting story, even with this typical *Mail* language, "the Nobel prize genius Crick was high on LSD when he discovered the secret of life." It's much more complicated than that, of course, and we know that Crick was in a sense involved in the plagiarism of others' work—there was a whole research background to the understanding of the DNA molecule. But he appears to have told someone at some time that he had perceived the double-helix shape while on LSD. I would suggest that if there's any truth to that—it is known that Crick was a regular user of LSD, and also a big advocate of ending the war on drugs, and good for him for doing that—then it was in an LSD experience or through an LSD experience that he managed to integrate what he knew and that it did play a role in the discovery of the double helix.

So are all the different techniques and substances for altering consciousness really portals to other worlds and dimensions—which shamans believe and some scientists believe—from where we return with novelty, with news, and with stuff we didn't know before and implement it into human culture? That's why I subtitled my book *Meetings with the Ancient Teachers of Mankind.* Or could there be some other explanation?

I will just float this explanation rapidly; it isn't one that I particularly favor, but it's interesting. Is it possible—this is what quite a lot of scientists would say—that these experiences are in some sense hardwired into the human brain and that this is why they are transpersonal and universal, like other aspects of human behavior? It does appear that there are hardwired brain modules. We all have intuitive physics, everybody can do incredible calculations without even knowing they're doing them, so if I throw a paper ball at you, if you are alert you'll sweep it aside and it won't hit you; you can see why evolution would invest in modules like that. If you didn't have rock-dodging genes, you'd be less likely to pass them on to your offspring than if you did have them.

But why would there be a brain module, why would millions of years of evolution equip the entire human race with brain modules for therianthropes and abductions by spirits and fairies and aliens? Why should these spirit molecules only be activated in altered states of consciousness? What use could they possibly be?

So we come back to Francis Crick and his really rather extraordinary book called *Life Itself,* which he published in 1981 and is all about DNA, really the DNA–RNA system. Crick was an advocate of directed panspermia, along with Sir Fred Hoyle. The bottom line of the argument was that it's been 13 billion years since the Big Bang. There's been time for life to have evolved more than once in the universe. He hypothesized that an alien civilization in a distant galaxy, which had achieved a high level of development, discovered that it was going to be utterly destroyed by some cosmic accident, perhaps a supernova explosion in the vicinity or something like that. Their first thought, he proposed, would be to get themselves off the planet and start their project again somewhere else.

But they would find that the laws of physics limited those possibilities, the vast distances of interstellar space. So he then suggested maybe what they'd do is genetically engineer bacteria to make them extremely resistant, pack them into cryogenic chambers and then put them on rockets and fire them off into the universe in all directions. Crick's explanation for the origin of life on Earth, at least as he expresses it in *Life Itself,* is that one of those spaceships hit the early Earth 3.8 billion years ago and spilled out its contents of bacteria, which immediately began reproducing and evolving. And 3.8 billion years later here we are, the end result of that process.

In other words: it was aliens.

If we take Crick's idea a little bit further, that the seeds of life have come here—the other option is panspermia, where they come on comets—as a *directed* process and that an attempt was made to send the seeds of life out into the universe, might they not have attempted to send something else as well? I'm not going to even attempt to explain the whole DNA thing to this room full of experts, you all know it already, but the interesting distinction is between coding and noncoding DNA and the whole problem of junk DNA, which is no longer regarded as junk by any serious researcher. I was struck by this paper from Eugene Stanley, who found a structure in noncoding DNA that was identical to the structure in all human languages that's to do with the relationship between frequency and rank, whereas in the coding regions of DNA that make proteins you get a different pattern than in the noncoding regions, but the latter is the same pattern that you get in all human languages. I rang up Stanley and asked him about this, and I had quite a long chat with him; and at the end of it I said, "So what's the bottom line, what do you think's going on?" And he said, "I think there's a message written in our DNA."

I don't know if he still holds to that, as I haven't talked to him since then. This raises an intriguing possibility with Crick's hypothesis, because we now know that DNA is a very effective storage medium—songs and books have already been recorded in DNA.

If our DNA originated elsewhere as a result of genetic engineering, what would there be to stop that hypothetical distant civilization from encoding information into the DNA? Perhaps that's what we're all universally accessing in altered states of consciousness: not a hidden doorway but a hidden archive within our own bodies that contains all the knowledge and all the information of an ancient and alien civilization.

I prefer the notion of freestanding parallel realms, which we are able to access through our consciousness with the aid of facilitators like DMT. But whether it's that or something else, it's clear that these substances are not in any sense brain candy. If used in the right way—responsibly with a focus on ensuring the most powerful effect—then they can be utterly transformatory, and we are indeed confronted by a tremendous mystery, as Dennis [McKenna] put it the other day.

It seems bizarre, you know, that our society will send us to prison and literally ruin our lives for making use of these time-honored sacred plants to explore our own consciousness and perhaps reconnect with spirit as our Stone Age ancestors did thirty-five thousand years ago. Surely this project of exploring the miracle and the mystery of our own consciousness is just about the most important thing possible for human beings to do. To deliberately limit human consciousness to a very narrow band and surround it with legislation may prove to be a very costly mistake. It could cost us the next step forward in our own evolution, I think. With reverence, with respect, and with serious intent, we should welcome the chance that our allies the plants are offering us: to explore the whole of reality and to discover our place within it.

DISCUSSION OF

Psychedelics, Entities, Dark Matter, and Parallel Dimensions

DAVID LUKE: Thank you, Graham. You covered a lot of ground there with your wonderful book *Supernatural,* and your talk, as a very condensed version of that work, was superb. This is more of a technical niggle really, but it was about the use of the term "entoptic" from Lewis-Williams . . .

GRAHAM HANCOCK: Within the eye, within the optic system.

LUKE: Yes, as in within the visual system, somewhere between the eye and the visual cortex. That in itself is an assumption, and we should progress from as few assumptions as possible.

HANCOCK: I completely agree with you.

LUKE: Okay, good. So Klüver, who did the original mescaline research looking at these patterns, called them "form constants," which is a more neutral term. I wrote a paper on this, and if you look at the kinds of experiences people talk about, particularly on DMT, when they're seeing these geometric patterns—let's call them form constants—often people report seeing them with more than three spatial dimensions; that's what they say, that they have extra dimensions. I asked Rick about this because there was a question on his Hallucinogen Rating Scale as to how many dimensions the visual percept had. There was three-dimensional, four-dimensional, extra-dimensional, and that kind of thing, and he said, from memory, all of the high-dose participants reported four or more spatial dimensions to these form constants. I think even explaining three-dimensional visual percepts based on the optic system is problematic because some miracle happens there. As for extra-dimensional percepts, why should we assume these originate somewhere in the optic system?

HANCOCK: I think it's a very misleading term; but it's there in literature, so I use it. The only thing that really intrigues me about the term is the universality of these experiences.

JILL PURCE: I'd just like to add a comment about those images of grids and chains. In Tibetan Buddhism the practice of *thögal* and the practices of the dark, where you spend forty-nine days in complete darkness in order to, as they say, allow the inner light and the external light to meet, patterns of grids and chains are one of the key things that are seen. There's a temple under threat at the moment in Lhasa—one of the Dalai Lama's temples—that shows many meditating figures, and in the sky you see these grids, chains, and *thigles* which are little balls of light like soap bubbles. This imagery is very typical of the kinds of things that come through when meditating in darkness with complete absence of light or, alternately, when contemplating while looking just underneath the sun or looking at bright sources of lights, mirrors, and so on.

HANCOCK: So again in a sense they appear to result from an altered state of consciousness—meditation—that seems to be the universal factor that we need to get out of the alert, problem-solving state of consciousness and into other states of consciousness . . .

PURCE: For which they use the light or the absence of light.

GRAHAM ST. JOHN: Graham, I want to ask you about your advent into the world of fiction with your book *Entangled: The Eater of Souls*. It's sort of related here because I'm fascinated with how Rick Strassman's ideas have impacted popular culture. In your book—which I think is a fascinating advent in entheo-fiction, where entheogens become a means by which one experiences supernatural powers, telepathy, time travel, and so on—you have a fictional character by the name of Doctor Bannerman, who undertakes human research into DMT . . .

HANCOCK: That's Rick.

ST. JOHN: . . . and research into the sixth sense, so I just wonder if you could talk a little bit about that.

HANCOCK: So the first oddity was that I had never been a fiction writer; I had always written nonfiction. I was a journalist before I got into books, and nonfiction was my thing. I had this feeling going back to my childhood that I would like to write fiction, but I didn't feel confident about doing it, and I wasn't even sure what I wanted to write about. Just something, it was a vague wish that I made the focus of my intent at another series of sessions at Wasiwaska, probably in 2006 or 2007, where in a series of visions I was given the story that ended up being the essential bones of the story *Entangled*. I saw certain scenes, I saw the characters, I saw principally Ria and Leoni, the two women, and I saw the Neanderthals in a way I'd never seen them before.

Because when I wrote *Supernatural* I bought in to the knuckle-dragging Neanderthal image, and we all know now how much that image has changed in the last decade. I presented the Neanderthals as basically nonspiritual apes in *Supernatural*. I was shown a totally different aspect of Neanderthals in these experiences with ayahuasca, of a telepathic creature filled with love—quite a different story. So I was given inspiration definitely: I asked for it, I got it, and I was given a strong impulse to go away and write a book. So I did. That book was *Entangled,* and it was the first novel that I've written. And of course aspects of it are not the result of visions; aspects of it are the result of what I already know. And yes, I wanted a medical doctor who was doing research involving DMT and also near-death experiences, and that was the landscape in which it unfolded. And then I had to grapple with the whole issue of good and evil in that book—what that means and how it comes into the human domain.

St. John: When will we be able to read the completion of the second book?

Hancock: Probably not until the end of 2016, but I intend to finish it next year. It may be even 2017 until it comes out.

St. John: Thank you.

Jeremy Narby: Graham, I quibble with extending the term "shaman" and shamanism back tens of thousands of years . . .

Hancock: Fair enough.

Narby: . . . and, just briefly, what I think it obscures is something interesting. First of all, of course, the term "shaman" is a kind of a transcultural label that anthropologists have taken out of Siberia . . .

HANCOCK: Because it belongs to the Tungus Mongols . . .

NARBY: . . . and extended to hundreds of different cultures around the world. Then the question was, So how far back in time can we extend it? So now the question is, So what is it? You gave the definition of modified states of consciousness as being at the heart of what shamans do. Let's just take that: they do not leave fossils or physical traces so, actually, if you're strict with evidence, it's hard to demonstrate the prehistory of whether shamans were around. So then the idea with the cave art is that because obviously there is something going on that does seem to involve modified states of consciousness, that the caves themselves were facilitating modified consciousness and that going into them was the equivalent of working. So it was that humans might at that point have been in the kind of kindergarten phase of learning what was later going to become what we now call shamanism—seventeen thousand years ago they were doing this—because modern-day shamans do not go into caves and paint them.

HANCOCK: No, you're right, that was something very much of that time, for some reason. Yes, I think the caves were a technique for altering consciousness, the perfect environment for sensory deprivation, where once you get inside you're cut off from the everyday realm in lots of ways.

PURCE: You know there's some evidence that the caves chosen were chosen because of the extreme resonance?

HANCOCK: Yes. The sound effects were stunning in the painted caves—that's the way the sounds work—and that's true in a number of ancient monuments as well, places like the Great Pyramid, which also has very powerful sound aspects. Yes, again it's a short cut. I can't prove that these people were ritual functionaries of the kind that we now call shamans. All I can say is that in their art they are manifesting evidence for altered states of consciousness, and that is, I would say, the central aspect of shamanism. I don't think that anybody who would be referred to as a shaman would be practicing without an altered state of consciousness being involved in some way, but it might be induced by all kinds of different techniques.

VIMAL DARPAN: We do have the evidence in Australia of an unbroken line of fifty thousand years of aboriginal, for want of a better word, shamanism, where in fact that person—the *karadji,* or "Cleverman"— has always been there, fifty thousand years ago just as he is in modern-day times. So one could infer from a living indigenous culture of that age that perhaps that might have been extended fifty thousand years ago in the European continent as well.

HANCOCK: Interesting point. The curious thing for me, coming from this whole body of research that I and many others have been involved in, is that these three supposedly different categories of beings—spirits, fairies, and aliens, at the level of phenomenology—all appear to be the same thing. This then carries the entity encounter, which we are all mystified by today, back deep into prehistory. Because of at least the correlation between altered state of consciousness art and a big jump forward in the evolution of human behavior, we should want to know more about this. This is the question we're all here to examine: are there real entities, real realms, underneath us? Or it's almost as incredible that it would all be made up in the human mind and actually made up the same way by human minds all over the world. I think it's a fascinating problem and a rich area for future inquiry.

ANTON BILTON: I have a query. Among the many commonalities of the entity experience, the one that sort of shines forth is that they seem more intelligent; they are running the show . . .

HANCOCK: They're definitely running the show.

BILTON: . . . when we bump into them, and in terms of their nature, sometimes it's wonderful and divine, but many times it's ambivalent;

one's not quite sure what they're up to or why they're giving us the interest that they do. In some ways it's not dissimilar to a farmer with his sheep, you know: I'm going to look after the herd, and I'm going to check their teeth, and I'm going to probe around and make sure they don't die. My question is, Are they the farmer and are we the sheep?

AUDIENCE MEMBER: Are we the food?

BILTON: Are we being farmed and at death our souls are devoured in some way?

HANCOCK: Or how about this: that the realm we call physical—the physical world, our world, the earth that we live on—maybe it's a creation of a nonphysical realm? Maybe. This is pure speculation, of course. We don't know what consciousness is. We feel it must have a physical or a biological substrate because it does in our case, but perhaps not. But if you're in a realm of pure consciousness where there's no physicality, then it's difficult to learn and it's difficult to have experiences.

BILTON: You can imagine if one's running the show and looking down on a weaker species, the one thing one would proffer is goodness, if you like. So if there's a sinister or observational aspect, you wonder why the goodness isn't flowing through. "Hello, we've found a new race, welcome," as opposed to this ambivalent and somewhat mechanical mentality to our relationship.

HANCOCK: I completely agree with you about the ambivalent nature of the entities and the fact that there are encounters with what feels like pure evil in those realms from time to time . . .

BILTON: Good farmers and bad farmers.

HANCOCK: The good farmer and the bad farmer—you know I've been involved in sessions where that has happened. I've seen numbers of people affected as if there were something flying around the room, hitting different people in different ways. There was a particular session, again at Wasiwaska, where one of the participants had an encounter with the entity that we tend to construe as Mother Ayahuasca, and Mother Ayahuasca said she'd had to show him that because that was the only way that he could understand what she has to deal with all the time. In a sense, if these are entities, they aren't actually powerful in the physical realm; they can only leverage the physical realm through affecting consciousness. And maybe some of them have very unpleasant motives. It's possible; I don't rule that out at all.

RICK STRASSMAN: I think it's important to distinguish the quality of the beings that we encounter. In my new work, I discuss the similarities between beings encountered in the DMT state and angels in the Hebrew Bible. It is possible to distinguish, at least in the Hebrew Bible and I think in shamanism as well, between lying spirits, demons, angels, and various other entities that are positive, negative, and somewhere between. There need to be some criteria and tests that we can apply to these beings to determine their nature, some yardsticks for being either benign or malign. That's where I think some of the Jewish, Christian, and Muslim teachings can help to differentiate and utilize the differences between the various levels of beings because it can be quite hard to discern. It makes all the difference in the world if we're taking advice, or allowing something to work on us that's bad or good. Those are some of the issues that I think are critical in determining the value of who we're dealing with or what we're dealing with.

HANCOCK: I absolutely agree. I mean it's like an exploration of a strange land we don't know: Some of the inhabitants may be very loving and positive and want the best for strangers that visit their lands, and others might be quite the opposite—psychic vampires or parasitical predators of some kind. It would be really good to know what we're dealing with, and that's again a reason for vastly expanding the scientific research into this field.

ANDREW GALLIMORE: I just want to make the point that perhaps the DMT world is populated by beings that created us. Now, in my talk I spoke very briefly about the simulated universe idea, and I think "the world is a computer simulation" is perhaps an oversimplification, but it's an interesting starting point. Engineer Brian Whitworth, who's written a lot about simulated universe theory, points out, I think quite pertinently, that the simulator reality, the reality that's doing the simulating, must have at least one more dimension than the simulated reality; and what's interesting of course is that that would mean that the brain is a three-dimensional projection of a higher-dimensional processor, and with appropriate reprogramming—when DMT is ingested—the brain might be able to process and render higher-dimensional data. Hence, higher-dimensional entoptics—impossible objects with four, five, six dimensions—that might explain it.

HANCOCK: Interesting.

LUKE: It's worth asking Bernard, I think, if it's possible that the extra dimensions observed in the DMT realm might be explained by M theory, for example.

BERNARD CARR: I hadn't heard about Brian Whitworth until you mentioned him. I think Graham referred, in some remark earlier, to the possibility of seeing higher-dimensional geometries. I'm not completely clear how one actually analyzes the dimensionality of the object you're seeing from a mathematical perspective, but to me that is the obvious test of hyperspatial models of these experiences, seeing things which are not possible in a normal three-dimensional world. But I have no expertise in the actual experience.

HANCOCK: Andrew, this morning you were talking about drip feeding DMT and the possibility of a group of volunteers who might be sent on, I don't know, a one-week DMT trip?

GALLIMORE: Yes.

HANCOCK: If such a group of hardy adventurers could be discovered and brought together and were willing to go there—Luis will do it!—I would like to ask you, What would you task them with first? Would you task them at all? Would you say we want you to look for something there, or . . . ?

GALLIMORE: I guess the most obvious thing I could think of—and you might disagree—is when you first enter a new territory, the first thing you would do as an ecologist or a biologist would be to sample the fauna and the flora. Perhaps the fauna might be more interesting to catalog, because of the various beings. I might task them with establishing communication perhaps, and really the point would be, first of all, to find some beings that were willing to communicate and could communicate. Then, establish a means of returning; maybe once we can spend more time in that realm the beings might be able to offer ways for us to know how to return to the same place.

HANCOCK: Is there a category of data or information that could be brought back from that realm that would settle the matter and would say to us, yes, this reality is definitely freestanding?

LUKE: That is the really interesting question. I think this also bears relevance to the point you raised, Graham, that perhaps ancestrally we had altered states of consciousness appearing, obviously indicated by art, at the same time as culture advanced and civilization began, etcetera. So was that information being fed by these discarnate entities in some way? I think part of answering that question ties in with the same question you're asking, Andrew: How do we go about testing the ontology of these very entities themselves?

Now Marko Rodriguez put forward this proposal: you send the entities some really difficult math tasks that you don't have the answers to but which you can then verify. This is a great idea, but then it falls down when you know a little bit about the psychical research, which has been going on already for about 130 years with mediums, trying to establish the veracity of communications with discarnate entities known as "spirits of the dead." It falls down on the problem of what's called the "super-psi hypothesis," which is that if you garner some great information from an apparently discarnate source—information which you shouldn't know already and that can be verified—that ultimately it could just be some kind of telepathy or clairvoyance, which presents a problem because we don't know any limitations for telepathy or clairvoyance as we currently understand them. And that means you can never prove discarnate communications, currently, as it may just be psi; i.e., telepathy or clairvoyance.

GALLIMORE: So what is an orthodox scientist going to say, when you say, well, these beings gave us answers to mathematical problems, "Ah, that's just telepathy!"

[Audience laughter.]

ERIK DAVIS: That's a function of that category; it arises specifically in reaction to the spiritual, so part of the whole development of telepathy as a concept was precisely to tear down the "other," so for us it seems ridiculous, but at that point in time it really was offered as an alternative to spirits.

WILL ROWLANDSON: Do you know I find it quite odd that we're still slightly stuck on this issue of the ontological status. If we are entering any form of debate about "wow, were these guys really important to our history?" then we're going to also be asking if they are important to our history right now. And therefore if we're trying to shove things at them and say, "Do this mathematical sum; let me pick a flower from your garden," we're kind of missing a bit of the point, which is just sitting down and talking. That's what I feel. Sorry.

LUKE: No, I totally agree, you're right. I think that's all well and good for us here in this room, who perhaps take a bit more of an open view about it, but for the rest of the research community and the academic world, and the world at large, perhaps, they may well ask, "Can you actually give us some evidence of this, beyond the experience itself?"

ROWLANDSON: Evidence? I mean, what are you going to do? Bring back a bloody elf? I mean, I'm sorry, but I made this point. "I've caught an elf" is not going to happen. It's not.

NARBY: I want to return to the question that Rick brought out and comment that I appreciated the way that you started with your trip report. I thought it was very pertinent, and then I thought you were going to interpret it as meaning that these can be dangerous, dark places and that we should be more worried about going there and more prudent. But in fact, you didn't go there, and then your brilliant overview of the whole question was rather enticing, so I was left with a feeling of ambiguity.

HANCOCK: There is an ambiguity. The dark and terrifying experience, in the sense of an encounter with evil, is the most horrible experience that we can have in these states of consciousness. I actually haven't smoked pure DMT since that experience—I've smoked changa, but I haven't smoked pure DMT—and I'm hesitant to go back into that. It was a shocking experience for me. So the question is, you know, what are we dealing with here? What I observe is that the most troubling and most disturbing journeys, after a while, end up being the most useful ones. They're the ones that we really took something home from, we learned something about. I underwent a significant change in my habitual behavior following that experience, plus the five sessions of ayahuasca immediately afterward, in Wasiwaska. There's this notion in which a friend of mine describes this realm as a university of duality and that we are here in this physical form to experience the lessons that duality has to teach. Duality has to involve the dark and the light, the good and the evil. They're part of it, but in a sense it's possible to transcend it; there are lessons to learn in the physical realm, and they are lessons that are not for the fainthearted.

RICK STRASSMAN: Yes, I wanted to respond to the fellow who said, "Well, what do we do, bring back an elf?" You know I think that's probably a ways into the future, but . . . in the meantime I think it would be worthwhile to bring a high-level mathematician into the group and start working on establishing the mathematical possibility of bringing back an elf. You know, for example, some of Einstein's own theories were first developed clearly in his mind from mathematical models, and then only later—thirty, forty, fifty years—was there empirical data backing up his mathematical models. So if it's possible to find a sympathetic mathematician to work out some mathematical models to substantiate the possibility of bringing back an elf, I think that would lay the groundwork for future empirical work.

GALLIMORE: Well, I just think, could you ask the elves for the spatial coordinates in a binary form or something such that we could 3D print an elf?

HANCOCK: That's lateral thinking!

[Lots of laughter and shouts.]

LUKE: The classic example of this problem was this great study published in the *Journal of the Society for Psychical Research*. A chess grand master was playing a game, via a medium, apparently with a previous chess grand master, now dead, and he was convinced. It was a high-level game, you can check out how sophisticated the chess game was in the published article, and he concluded that only a grand master, a previous one, would have been able to play chess at that level. So it "must" have been someone who was dead, because he was the greatest living chess grand master, and it was a medium who wasn't even a chess player ordinarily that was making the moves. So the researchers concluded, "There you go. This is evidence of the discarnate survival of bodily death" because this woman was channeling information from a discarnate chess grand master. But then somebody obviously pointed out, "Well, could she just have been getting the moves telepathically from the living guy she was playing with?" So how do we know what the source of the information is? Where is it coming from, if we have the possibility of telepathy, clairvoyance, or precognition?

HANCOCK: It's a very difficult problem to solve; it's a very challenging research problem actually in every way.

LUKE: But even then, if we do come out with some kind of new fantastic mathematical formula or perhaps a theory of everything—maybe we can task the elves to give us a theory of everything?

BILTON: What about the coordinates of a moon or star we don't know about yet, a little bit like a Sirius Dogon scenario? Give us something we don't know, and then we'll get a telescope or whatever and find it.

HANCOCK: That could work.

LUKE: I guess if you have something useful it's still something useful regardless of the source, but it doesn't specifically answer the ontological question, which is: How do we catch an elf?

HANCOCK: That appears to be what happened in the upper Paleolithic. Something useful was transferred, and there was a change in human behavior, which correlates with evidence of this kind of experience. It doesn't prove anything, but from time to time something new seems to come out of this. But then it may not be a teaching of information from nonphysical consciousnesses in another dimension; it could just be that psychedelics work on the brain in such a way that the brain becomes more effective at doing these things. I don't know.

LUKE: There are some excellent examples of great innovations and inventions that came from dreams, actually, from the invention of the sewing machine to [August] Kekulé's discovery of the benzene ring, and the mathematical formulas of the great Indian mathematician from last century, Ramanujan, who claimed his formulas were given to him in his dreams by discarnate entities.

HANCOCK: It's ironic in a way—within our culture if you call somebody a dreamer you're insulting them. It is one of the signs of the many problems with our culture.

Cosmo Feilding Mellen: I'm just wondering what you think about what Dennis [McKenna] was saying about it being Gaia and nature people are communing with, rather than it being aliens?

Hancock: Yes, every bit as strong an argument. The problem we have to explain is why there are these transpersonal experiences of encounters with entities. They are apparent today, and they also cross time, and they go back deep into the story of the human race. I think that's a really huge problem that needs to be explained. Right now we don't have an explanation for it. I'm suggesting something, Dennis was suggesting something else. In a sense the panspermia argument—the notion that the information was encoded in highly conserved sections of DNA a very long time ago—would answer Dennis's question: it could be an alien implant. It could be.

Purce: I'm just wondering if they give their name, like Rumpelstiltskin.

Hancock: If the entities give their names?

Purce: Or if people ask them their names.

Hancock: That's an interesting thought. I've never asked them their names. "Who are you?" I like that.

Purce: Who are they, and in whose name are they working?

Luis Luna: I think if the question is going to be, "Who are you?" The answer is, "We are you."

[Laughter.]

Luke: I think that rounds it off nicely. Thank you very much, Graham.

Hancock: A pleasure.

CHAPTER 10

The Nature of DMT Beings

Perspectives and Prospects

RICK STRASSMAN

Psychedelic drugs modify every aspect of consciousness: perception; mood and emotion; somatic or body sensations and awareness; mental processes, including production of novel content; and one's sense of self, volition, or will.

Let's briefly review some of the considerations in naming these substances. There are scientific versus popular terms to consider, as well as political correctness, and so on. Those inform nomenclature but accuracy is most important. Common terms are psychedelic, hallucinogen, entheogen, psychotomimetic, mind- or consciousness-expanding, psycho-integrator, empathogen, and entactogen.

I prefer *psychedelic* because it's the most generic. It means "mind-disclosing" or "mind-manifesting." It captures the fact that either nothing may happen or a lot may happen, and what happens may be good or bad. The major drawback to *psychedelic* is the accrued negative cultural associations that have attached to it over the decades.

The preferred medical-legal term is *hallucinogen,* meaning "generating hallucinations," but this is not accurate because visions and voices aren't invariant. It also begs the question of "what is a hallucination?"

It assumes that what we are experiencing is pathological and unreal, *a priori*.

"Entheogen" is a more popular term, but it's also limited because of its implicit assumption of the existence of divinity or spirituality. Can an atheist or a radical materialist have an entheogenic experience? Would Richard Dawkins want to take an entheogen? I think next time Graham [Hancock] challenges Richard Dawkins [to trip], it's important to make sure he uses the term "psychedelic." In addition, this term points to the source of divinity as within. This has yet to be established and is a theological, not psychological, assumption.

An older term is *psychotomimetic*. It is still used in some of the German literature. But apropos of "entheogen" for the atheist, who among us would want to take a "psychotomimetic"? In addition, what is psychosis? Even more than hallucinogen, this term judges the altered state as purely pathological.

Mind/consciousness-expanding also is too limited. What if your consciousness contracts? *Psycho-integrator* suffers from the same problem: What happens if your mind disintegrates? *Entactogen* or *empathogen* both emphasize putative beneficial psychological effects—"generating relatedness or empathy." However, the compounds usually referred to—MDMA and its congeners—are not classical psychedelics like LSD, psilocybin, mescaline, and DMT. It may be that low doses of the classical drugs are more like MDMA, but this hasn't been studied carefully yet in a head-to-head comparison using a within-subject design. It also suffers from similar limitations as the other terms; that is, people may feel cut off from themselves or from others rather than closer.

So we return to psychedelic. It's the most accurate term, and we should consider reclaiming it. There are a lot of words that have been misused—for example, *love* and *God*—but that doesn't mean we can't use them. It just requires we use greater precision and accuracy and are ready to defend their use. I think this is increasingly taking place in the scientific literature.

There are many fields that can be enriched by considering the psychedelic experience, and there are many fields that can enrich our understanding and application of the psychedelic experience. These include, among others, religion or spirituality, psychology, creativity, art, brain function, sociology, and even cosmology.

Today I'll be talking primarily religion and spirituality, and the strengths and the weaknesses they may bring to bear on the scientific study of the psychedelic state. There's a number of ways in which religion and spirituality address issues relevant to these substances' effects: the nature of invisible worlds, morality, foretelling, and revelation. The ones that I believe are relevant to this discussion are the Eastern religious—especially Buddhist—view on enlightenment, the shamanic model of controlling spiritual forces, and the prophetic experience in the Hebrew Bible or Old Testament.

Before going further, let me put several urban myths to rest. Even though I marshal what I believe is good circumstantial evidence, we don't yet know if endogenous DMT levels increase at birth or death; we don't know if DMT activity increases during nondrug DMT-like states, such as dream sleep, meditation, or alien contact; and we don't know if there's a difference in DMT activity in people with calcified pineal glands.

What do we know about DMT? The first wave of DMT research took place in the 1950s and 1960s, with the last studies completing in the early 1970s. The focus at that time was on psychotic illness, especially schizophrenia, in order to establish a role for endogenous DMT in the etiology of these illnesses. Research compared the phenomenology of the two states: the DMT state and the psychotic one. How similar were they? If very, then perhaps endogenous DMT might be involved in endogenous psychosis. They also compared DMT blood levels between normal subjects and schizophrenics. They tried to reduce DMT activity—either by blockading its effects or somehow inhibiting its formation—as putative antipsychotic treatments. They also decreased its breakdown with MAOIs [monoamine oxidase inhibitors] to see if psychotic symptoms worsened.

Our DMT study took place in the early 1990s. We studied almost five dozen normal volunteers, administering the drug intravenously. We completed three studies in five years. The first was a dose-response project where people got placebo and four different doses of drug: one small, two medium, and one high dose. We also did a second project to determine if tolerance developed in response to closely spaced repeated dosing. Tolerance—decreased effects with closely spaced repeated dosing—occurs with other psychedelics but hadn't been demonstrated with DMT. We thought it was a matter of shortening the interval enough, so we gave, in one morning, four fully psychedelic doses separated by half-hour intervals. Even then, we did not demonstrate tolerance to DMT's psychological effects. In our third project, we looked at the serotonin receptors mediating the drug effect. Over the course of five years, we gave about four hundred doses of varying strengths.

When a fully psychedelic dose of DMT is given, the effects begin within a couple of heartbeats. There's a rapidly building rush—inner tension and acceleration, anxiety or excitement—with an accompanying sound that gets louder and louder. The rush and sound climax with the sensation of a separation of the mind from the body. One enters into a world of bright light that is intensely saturated, rapidly morphing, buzzing, and moving. One's sense of self is maintained. It is usually intense emotionally but can also be relatively neutral emotionally, especially compared to the perceptual effects. The DMT "world" was described as "inhabited" by at least half of our volunteers, who reported some kind of sentient presence or presences with whom they interacted in this state. There was much give and take. Only rarely was the experience "unitive," where one's self dissolved into a timeless, spaceless, concept- and perception-free state.

This finding of interactions predominating over mystical unification was in contrast with what both my volunteers and I expected. The paradigmatic mystical-unitive experience, at least from what I had studied over the years, is the Zen kenshō, or "enlightenment experience," where one's sense of self dissolves into the ground of being, *sunyatta*—the Buddhist notion of "emptiness"—no perceptions, verbal content, or sense of self. It is the goal of kabbalah viz attaining *ein sof,* "no ending," as well as the goal of Christian mysticism. One might encapsulate the phenomenon by saying it's "being one with God."

However, the interactive-relational experience is what the volunteers in our study encountered. One's sense of self was maintained, one could willfully interact with the concept- and image-rich state. This is more akin to the prophetic experience described in the Hebrew Bible. Instead of "being one with God," one is "being with God," in an interactive relationship.

There seem to me to be two questions to address in discussions of the DMT world and its contents. One overarching question is, What is the nature of the DMT world; is it real or unreal? That segues into subquestions: Is it an inner or outer experience? Is it objective or subjective? The other major question is, If so, so what? That is, What is it good for? Other than our knowing that it's there, we need to consider whether the world is a better place, or we are better off, for knowing about it. This is where the meaning and the message of the state take precedence.

The first question deals with the reality of the DMT world. One of the caveats, maybe *the* caveat, of the real or unreal debate is the notion of DMT as the *endomatrix,* an endogenous substance or process that creates our apprehension of everyday reality. There are two pieces of data that confuse, or muddy, any facile distinctions between real and unreal. One is data generated by a Japanese group several decades ago, as well as a more recent Brazilian study. These studies demonstrated that DMT is transported into the brain across the blood-brain barrier using an energy-dependent process.

This treatment by the brain is characteristic of that substance being an essential brain nutrient. Other examples are glucose and certain amino acids the brain cannot synthesize on its own. That the brain expends energy in getting DMT into its confines suggests that DMT is required for normal brain function. And normal brain function means normal consciousness. This led me to consider DMT as a type of reality thermostat, where a narrow window of DMT levels in the brain maintains our sense of consensus reality. In addition, Nick Cozzi and his group in Madison, Wisconsin, recently demonstrated that the genetic machinery for DMT synthesis is active in the retina. Besides regulating general consciousness, it may be that DMT also regulates our perception of the visual world.

When speculating about mechanisms and mechanistic model building, one can divide these into the bottom-up and top-down categories. One bottom-up model is the brain biology model, or neurotheology, the reigning paradigm of the biology of spiritual experience. It posits that the DMT world is a manifestation of a brain on drugs—the DMT world is *generated* by the brain. And the brain is so configured in order to bestow evolutionary advantages to those members of a species having such experiences. Those evolutionary boons include, for example, creativity and altruism. However, neurotheology does not help us answer *why* DMT does those things. It only explains *how*. In other words, why do these results of selected psychedelic experiences on altruism and creativity bestow selective advantages? Why don't they bestow evolutionary disadvantages? In addition, this model posits that the DMT world is not objectively real.

The other bottom-up model is the psychological one, more specifically the psychoanalytic. This teaches that the DMT world is your mind on drugs. It is a product of your mind, the contents being symbolic representations of the unconscious. While these representations may provide leverage for psychotherapeutic change, they are not objectively real.

Even Zen Buddhism takes a bottom-up approach to explicating the nature of the DMT world. Other sects of Buddhism, for example the Tibetan and Theravada, may look at the contents of visionary states differently than Zen, but Zen was my spiritual scaffolding at the time I performed my studies and is one of the most influential Eastern religions to have set root in the West. Zen opines that the DMT world is your mind-brain complex on drugs. The visions and voices are mental detritus being shed on the way toward the formless, enlightened state, which is empty. It advises that the visions and the voices are best ignored, because they're distractions and not objectively real.

Top-down models posit the reality of the DMT world and its objective and freestanding nature. A secular Western version is what I tentatively settled on at the end of my first DMT book; that is, DMT changes the receiving characteristics of the mind-brain complex and allows us to peer into usually invisible worlds, much as a microscope does. These worlds are also of interest to modern physics and include such notions as dark matter and parallel universes. Due to DMT-induced brain changes, we may now be able to perceive the contents, including the inhabitants, of those worlds. This model provides a link to religious and spiritual models, in that the DMT world is now considered not simply to be a hallucination.

As I will describe, the Hebrew Bible's religious model—as opposed to "mind-only" Eastern models—is also top-down. It proposes that spiritual experiences are real apprehensions of externally existent levels of reality. Both top-down religious and the scientific models invoked to explain the nature of the DMT world share an interest in mechanisms of action—how we are able to perceive normally invisible levels of reality. However, they also diverge in their purview, in their charge.

One of the advantages of religious models is that they suggest why things are configured this way. Rather than random collections of molecules, there is a guiding organizing principle responsible for those collections, configured in that way for a purpose. For example, we are able to perceive normally invisible worlds because of God's configuring the brain that way—in order for us to understand things about God that are normally inaccessible. Things like providence, and natural and moral laws. This way religious models are a better framework for integration at personal and social levels. Religious models, while they are interested in mechanisms, are also interested in the messages, the information content, contained in these highly altered states. It is not a matter of simply describing and attempting to manipulate them. Therefore, religious models may be more relevant to those interested in using these drugs for religious or spiritual purposes.

Before going much further into Hebrew Bible theology and metaphysics, it's important to at least attempt to dispel knee-jerk antireligious reactions to what's coming next. This I will attempt by distinguishing between the straw man "religion" that many atheists like to trot out as their whipping boy and a more sophisticated view of religion, especially that which is contained within the Hebrew Bible.

The philosopher Spinoza distinguished between the religion of the masses—which he equated with superstition, which preys on fear and hope—and the religion of the elite or of the philosophers. The latter is more accurately characterized as love and knowledge of God, something one attains through the prophetic state or through scientific inquiry. One can attain an understanding of natural and perhaps moral law experimentally, but this can be done more quickly through true prophetic experience.

With that as a prelude, let's look at the contemporary religious models for the psychedelic state in general and the DMT one in particular.

I've discussed the Zen Buddhist approach. Its two drawbacks are that the DMT state isn't like enlightenment, it's more interactive than unitive. And Zen posits that the things apprehended in that state are unreal.

Latin American ayahuasca shamanism has the advantages of positing the reality of the contents of the state, but it has ethical and moral challenges. These, I think, are related to its fundamentally occult nature, in which primacy is granted to manipulating spiritual forces for one's own purposes.

Both the Zen and shamanic models, in addition, are foreign. They do not resonate with the Western mind, at conscious and unconscious levels, as much as a model that is garbed in more culturally relevant images and concepts. I believe that any model that's going to get any traction among the most people in the West needs to be made as palatable and as familiar as possible. The psychedelic worlds are so strange in the first place that if they can be presented in terms that people can relate to, using notions and vocabulary common to the Western mind, it may be easier to penetrate, be seen as more applicable, and lead to wider-ranging discussions and applications.

The nature of the DMT world requires that any model be interactive-relational, because that's what the DMT state is. It also must posit that the DMT state is as real as or more real than everyday reality—a nearly universal description of the DMT state by my volunteers and most in-the-field users.

This second criterion—accepting the reality of other worlds—came about from my experience beginning the DMT study. I entered the project armed with bottom-up models such as: the DMT world is the brain on drugs—what we might called neurotheology—the DMT world is a Zen Buddhist delusion, and from psychology it is the unconscious on steroids. All rest on the assumption that what people are experiencing on DMT is "something else," it's not really what they just experienced. Quickly, I found that this approach did not encourage people to share some of the most interesting, and oftentimes unsettling, aspects of their drug sessions. At a certain point I engaged in a thought experiment, saying to myself, "I will act as if people just entered into an alternative level of reality." What would be the results of such an experiment? Where do you go from there? How can that help us explicate what people are undergoing? Once I stopped subtly challenging the existential or ontological basis of what people were describing, a good flow of communication resumed.

Another criterion for a strong model is that it addresses ethical and moral, as well as theological, concerns. This could include a theistic worldview, in order that it appeal to the Western mind. These criteria all exist within a model articulated in the Hebrew Bible—the prophetic state.

Now, this will require a nontrivial degree of open-mindedness on your part, so please put on your open-minded caps. There is a natural aversion to the Hebrew Bible carried by most secular educated

Westerners. Nevertheless, one of the supposed hallmarks of being duly psychedelicized is being open-minded. Therefore, try to take off your anti-Bible, anti-God, and anti-Israel caps, at least for a while, in order to allow as much of this information as possible to at least register.

The Hebrew Bible is a collection of twenty-two books, written mostly in biblical Hebrew. It's not kabbalah, which is a centuries-later development that owes its existence to Christian and Eastern thought making its way into Judaism. The Hebrew Bible is the foundational religious text for half of the planet's population. It influences all of civilization: economics, theology, architecture, aesthetics, politics, sociology, anthropology, medicine, ritual, morality, and ethics. It's clearly powerful, and its power exerts influence wherever we turn. It's been in circulation for at least two thousand five hundred years, and there's no reason why it should be closed to, or spurned by, the psychedelic community. It's not reasonable that only certain people—many of whom are unscrupulous in their use of its power—have access to the text.

There are many resistances to reading the text—emotional and intellectual. Concepts like God, reward and punishment, commandments, creation, Israel, and so on can make it seem incomprehensible. This is why we need commentaries, the most useful of which were written by authors between the turn of the Common Era and the thirteenth century.

There are other ways to break down those resistances. You can read the text out loud, which is especially effective if done in Hebrew. Nevertheless, there are good English translations that, if read out loud, are also quite powerful in establishing resonance between you and the text. Intense study leads to an altered state, which resonates with the state out of which the text emerged—the prophetic state. Here, the commentators are the sitters, supportively explaining to you what it is you're reading and providing a comforting presence while you're floundering in the text.

The paradigmatic spiritual experience in the Hebrew Bible is prophecy. I define this as any spiritual experience occurring in any figure described in the text. It doesn't necessarily have to be a canonical prophet like Isaiah. And it is any spiritual experience, not only those that include foretelling or prediction. The association between foretelling and prophecy is an artifact of the Greek translation of the Hebrew word for prophet, *navi,* which the Greeks translated as *prophetes,* "one who speaks before something happens." The Greeks were interested in the divinatory properties of religious experience and their utility in predicting or divining. However, navi, the Hebrew word for prophet, means "an interpreter or translator, a spokesperson."

The Hebrew Bible is an account of prophetic experience, composed and edited by those in a prophetic state; thus it's a prophetic text. That, I believe, is the source of the power of the Bible. It's similar to when you read the Buddhist sutras. The sutras are verbal descriptions of the enlightened state, and reading them is quite compelling. In the case of the Hebrew Bible, it's a prophetic text, or verbal descriptions of the prophetic experience, which is equally compelling in its own way.

Let's look at Ezekiel chapter 1. In Ezekiel's initial theophany, the heavens opened, he saw visions of God, there was a stormy wind, a great cloud flashing fire, brilliance surrounding it, lightning, and a semblance of beings emerged from the midst of the fire. There are spheres, wheels. Ezekiel sees faces of beings: a man, lion, ox, and eagle. The beings run rapidly to and fro despite the immobility of their legs. The beings' backs and wings are full of eyes. Some beings fly through space, controlled by other beings. The sound of wings is like great rushing waters. There is an expanse of blue, or a rainbow, over the beings' heads. Ezekiel is overwhelmed, loses all strength, and falls on his face. An angel stands him up, speaks to him, pulls him by the hair, and carries him through space.

This complex vision of Ezekiel is called by the rabbis the "chariot." This is an example of what I call "the equivalence of imagery." One uses the available repertoire of mental imagery, the imaginative constituents, to garb or clothe the information contained in the visions. It may have looked like a chariot to Ezekiel, but it may look like a lab, or a UFO, or a futuristic landscape to modern secularists. However, equivalence of imagery suggests that the same information is contained in the different images and could be extracted with the proper interpretive keys.

Struck by similarities between descriptions by my volunteers of the DMT state and the reports of prophetic experience in the Hebrew Bible, I began comparing the two syndromes' phenomenology. If there was significant similarity, it would be legitimate to consider DMT as mediating prophetic phenomenology. My default mode for this comparison was the Buddhist Abhidharma psychological model of the *skandhas*. This is the system I had used to develop the rating scale for quantifying the DMT experience. These are the familiar concepts: form, feeling, perception, consciousness, understanding, and habitual tendencies. I morphed these into more traditional mental status and psychiatric terminology.

Once I began this comparison of the two states, I found that the overlap was striking. One of the areas of less than perfect overlap between the DMT and prophetic states hinges on the issue of the spoken voice versus the telepathic voice. If we assume that most of what prophetic figures hear in the text is telepathic rather than an outside voice, then this problem disappears. If we are looking for a spoken voice, then we would probably need to look at other endogenous compounds that elicit this phenomenon, such as the anticholinergic compounds.

While the degree of overlap was impressive, it seemed as if there was something missing in my categories, in that something was going on in the prophetic state that wasn't as well developed in the DMT one. This turned out to be a category I termed "relatedness," the nature of the interactions between the beings and those perceiving them. The interactions are primarily verbal but also work through other modalities such as the body, emotions, visual imagery, and sound. The primary function of relating was to communicate information.

There are a number of gradations in the level of intimacy in the relationship. One can be minimally engaged and just observe what's going on, or one can be minimally observed by the beings. One can overhear conversations among the beings. These examples occur both in the prophetic and the DMT experiences. Then there is more direct communication taking place: being spoken to by a being or speaking to a being. There can be two-way conversation, or there can be multiple parties involved in almost a group conversation.

One of the advantages attendant to a verbal model, as exemplified by the Hebrew Bible's prophetic one, is the ability to engage in enhanced interactions with the beings. One possesses words with which to communicate with the beings—and each other afterwards—in a way that may only be hinted at or alluded to in the perceptual and emotional components of the psychedelic experience. For example, there is ineffable, and then there is *ineffable*—there are varying degrees of ineffability. If we can approximate the experience 98 percent but not 100 percent, we are much further ahead than 0 percent, throwing up our hands in despair, saying that "there are just no words for it." The verbal currency also engages our intellect with the information contained in the state, and that intellectual engagement may be fruitfully pursued by studying the prophetic text. We can think about it, and exercise our intellects in attempting to understand, integrate, and communicate it, rather than simply attempting to remember and evoke inarticulate feelings and perceptions.

There is much more verbal information in the Hebrew Bible's characterization of the content of the prophetic experience than in the DMT state. But when the two do address the same issues, there is relatively good overlap—such as the existence and nature of the one God and the Golden Rule. There are also differences. In the DMT state, there were cases of volunteers helping, healing, guiding, or benefiting the beings. For example, someone transferred emotional energy and love to the beings who lacked them. Another volunteer found that she had to be careful how much she focused on the beings or how she asked questions, because they would shy away.

In general, the level of interaction and the depth and breadth of the data or information contained in the prophetic literature is significantly greater than that which most people bring back from the DMT experience. This leads one to consider whether the text of the Hebrew Bible, which is a spiritual text describing a DMT-like world, might help us extract information from the DMT state. And if you start looking at the prophetic message, this focuses primarily on the nature of reality, both spiritual and material, and how to relate to it in the highest possible manner: the least harm and the most good. These are key concerns to many of us who value the psychedelic state for its longer-term social and individual boons.

So we have "prophecy meets the DMT state." They're both interactive-relational rather than mystical-unitive. They both are experienced and believed to be more real than everyday reality. They are full of beings. And the prophetic text is accompanied by highly complex and far-reaching verbal descriptions of the message of the experience.

As a result of my Hebrew Bible research, I developed a new model, a top-down *theoneurological*. It brings God into the discussion and lays out a higher level of abstraction regarding why things are the way they are. It also may be useful in extracting more meaning from our psychedelic experiences. For example, neurotheology's answer as to why humans are constructed to have spiritual experiences is: because of their evolutionarily advantageous effect. In contrast, theoneurology answers: because this provides a means for God to communicate with us. It integrates theological plus materialistic models, hopefully combining the best rigor and wisdom of both. It's based on a contemporary treatment of medieval metaphysics developed by the Jewish philosophers. In particular, I'm indebted to Maimonides, who lived in Egypt around the 1200s. If one were to name his metaphysics, it would be called Neoplatonic Aristotelianism.

The medievalists basically suggest—and I use the word *basically* tongue in cheek because it took me years to distill what Maimonides and his heirs proposed—that there is a process of divine overflow, or emanation, from an incorporeal and categorically incomprehensible God. This God created and sustains cause and effect—the wheels that drive natural and moral law. This God existed before, and will exist after, cause and effect.

Emanation or divine efflux or overflow is carried by what are called "separate intelligences" by Aristotle and by the Jewish philosophers "intermediaries" or "angels." Intermediaries may be the most easily accepted term. These intermediaries regulate the spheres, field-like repositories of energy and information through which godly influence is exerted. The nature of this energy and information becomes increasingly coarse as one descends through them. These intermediaries are semicorporeal or quasi-material, as [Ede] Frecska mentioned yesterday. The last and coarsest sphere is the "sublunar," in which exists the earthly realm. The first of the intermediaries is sometimes called Metatron, or the first angel. However, I think this could also be conceived of as the Big Bang. It's the first manifestation of some "thing" that we can at least begin to comprehend, rather than some "thing"—God—that existed before the Big Bang, which, due to the absence of time and space as we know them, is incomprehensible.

The prophetic state devolves from divine overflow through the spheres—regulated by the intermediaries—onto one's equally and highly developed imaginative and rational faculties. The rational faculty extracts meaning from the divinely derived contents displayed in the imagination. By "imaginative faculty," I don't mean imaginary, as in made up, but rather the arena of the mind that contains the phenomenology—feelings, perceptions, and so on. Then the intellect extracts the meaning from those imaginative contents. Those imaginative contents may be verbal, but they still require the intellect to decipher, extract meaning, and interpret them.

It's interesting to note that the highest grade of prophecy was allegedly attained by Moses. Except for his initial epiphany, or theophany, at the burning bush, Moses experienced his prophetic communications nearly entirely verbally. He had almost no visions after the burning bush. In others' prophetic experiences detailed in the Hebrew Bible, occurring in non-Mosaic figures, there is always a measure of visionary experience.

Where does the information contained in the prophetic experience come from? Is it contained in the overflow? Or is it contained within us and the overflow only strengthens our capacities to access it? In either case, the information itself, or the new ability to perceive the information, comes from an outside source.

Theoneurology suggests that God created the brain in such a manner as to be able to communicate with us. This is in contrast to the neurotheology model, which suggests that the brain creates the *impression* of God communicating with us. In contrast, I propose that elevated activity of endogenous DMT may mediate the DMT-like features of the prophetic experience. I'm suggesting endogenous rather than exogenous DMT because there is no textual evidence for the mind-altering use of plants—other than grape wine—in the Hebrew Bible. Even if one were to agree with Benny Shanon's thesis that Moses's burning bush was a DMT-emitting *Acacia*, this was one isolated incident. It does nothing to explain 99.99 percent of other visionary or prophetic states in the text.

How does one go about experiencing prophecy? First, it is necessary to be qualified, an idea I will tie in to my later discussion of an enlarged definition of psychedelic. Being "qualified" means that one is capable of understanding what is apprehended in the prophetic state. The intellect can be trained through study. The medievalists recommended the classical disciplines: art, the sciences, grammar, music, and scripture. And learning and practicing ethical behavior keep the emotional mind free of degrading influences.

With respect to the imagination, its function may be enhanced via psychedelics. There are techniques that may *theoretically* enhance the activity of endogenous DMT—techniques that occasion DMT-like experiences such as fasting, prayer, sleep deprivation, and so on. These provide a richer soil for the planting of visionary experience.

When one possesses equally and highly developed imaginative and intellectual faculties, then one is "qualified." However, the ultimate arbiter for the attainment of prophecy is God. This caveat makes it impossible to force the issue. For example, one may be qualified, but

God will determine that the place, time, need, and community receptivity are suitable to bestow prophecy. There is also the notion that God may make one qualified miraculously in order to communicate at a particular time and place, in the absence of anyone already qualified. We thus see that being qualified and God having the final decision are dynamic concepts that interact with each other.

Does prophecy still exist? The rabbis declared an end to prophecy around the time of the Common Era. It's hard to imagine a biological mechanism despite Julian Jaynes's theories of structural or functional changes in the brain in response to particular social and climactic pressures. The rabbis' spiritual explanation—the miracle of withholding prophecy from qualified individuals—quickly gets convoluted. I think the more salient explanation is political. The Romans occupying Judea were intolerant of any politically disruptive individuals, which is by definition the role of the canonical prophet. In addition, Christianity was just beginning, so there was a rabbinic need to close off the prophetic canon and thus the prophetic lineage, denying prophetic status to Jesus and his followers. Despite the official declaration, if you look carefully at the Judaic stream since that time, the prophetic experience never really disappeared. Rather, it was marginalized and made more esoteric; for example, in kabbalah and Hasidism.

What is the prophetic message? Simply put, it is ethical monotheism. There is one God who revealed through prophecy the Golden Rule: love your fellow as yourself. The goal is world peace, not individual enlightenment or happiness. In this way, it significantly differs from the Eastern model.

Even though these two basic tenets of the prophetic message—one God and the Golden Rule—are relatively simple, at least verbally, they extend into every aspect of reality: social psychology, how to wage war, economics, the nature of the family, inheritances, and agriculture. In the latter case, the sabbatical laws instruct us to let fields lie fallow every seven years. Interestingly, there are no technological themes, such as how to build interstellar spacecraft or generate unlimited clean energy.

The Hebrew Bible also teaches by narrative and law the existence and nature of cause and effect; that is, if you don't follow the revealed guidelines for behavior and belief leading to social and individual health, there are consequences. For example, the ecological devastation that we are now seeing may be analogized to the "land vomiting out its inhabitants," described as the consequence of not following the Golden Rule and devotion to and belief in one God. In fact, one of the reasons the Hebrews were exiled from their land was because of their not following the law of the sabbatical.

There is a very interesting notion in the Hebrew Bible of the "world to come." If you look carefully at it, the world to come appears to be an incorporeal world with DMT-like features. And since I like coming up with wide-ranging, barely believable ideas—that, nevertheless, are at least potentially empirically testable—it's fascinating to speculate about a biological mechanism ushering in the world to come. Perhaps it represents or is the end result of the simultaneous activation of the genetic apparatus for DMT synthesis in all organisms possessing it. This would be a "biology of the rapture."

What would be the trigger, the stimulus, for this simultaneous widespread DMT event? One possibility is exogenous: some kind of celestial event such as a massive gamma burst. Or something endogenous: a genetic clock that is ticking in all of us. Or our own genetic engineering, say, of a highly contagious virus containing the promotor of the transcription of the DMT-synthesizing gene. Relevant to the "end of days," there's a phrase in Isaiah where God describes the onset of the world to come: "In its time I will hasten it." In other words, it will occur sooner or later, either from an external or internal stimulus.

One of the implications of the theoneurological model is that the Hebrew Bible may inform our thinking about the psychedelic state and its integration into our own and the larger world. For example, we might be able to learn how to interact more effectively with the beings by seeing how prophetic figures in the text did so. There's an episode in Joshua's career where he's confronted by an angelic being holding a sword. He doesn't know if it's a good or a bad being. He simply asks, "Are you with us, or against us?"

We also can apply biblical concepts, vocabulary, and narratives to the psychedelic state. Are we seeing one aspect or another of God? By entering into the psychedelic state with enhanced cognitive tools, we may be able to, for example, tailor our prayers using some of the blueprints laid out in the text. We would then be more ideally situated to pray in the most appropriate manner: petitioning, praising, or thanksgiving.

We can reclaim Western spirituality using the imaginative effects of psychedelics combined with the cognitive scaffolding of the Hebrew Bible. For example, The Zendo Project helps those at music festivals suffering from adverse effects of psychedelic drugs. A *zendo* is a Zen meditation hall. But what does a zendo have to do with psychedelics? Well, everything, if you look inside any contemporary head shop. Buddhas, incense, Tibetan bells, *dorjes,* and *thangkas.* One benefits from being contemplative and attentive, but why can't this resource be called The Tabernacle Project or The Temple Project? We are mindlessly appropriating an Eastern model for the psychedelic drug state without knowing very much about the nature and benefits of the Western one. It is unthinking and uncritical. Because of the resonance with our own Western spirituality—which may even extend down to the biological level; for example, relative abundance or sensitivity to DMT versus 5-methoxy-DMT and the different effects occasioned by each—we may benefit more using models that partake of Western spirituality than those that partake of New Age, shamanic, or Eastern models.

This adoption of an Eastern unitive-mystical paradigm is an even thornier, and thus studiously avoided, issue in the research community. Research projects take as a given that the unitive-mystical state is the goal of psychedelic experiences in both therapeutic and "clinical spirituality" projects. It is placed in front of volunteers, established as the goal, and drug sessions are steered in that direction. Correlations are made between the unitive-mystical state and the desired outcomes.

This is a trend beginning with Vivekananda's odyssey to the United States in the late 1800s, and we have yet to shine the light of day on it. Have we really determined that the Eastern unitive-mystical state is better, more to be sought after, helpful, or therapeutic than the interactive-relational one? Psychiatric researchers with minimal familiarity with religious studies claim that all religions value the mystical state. However, there is nothing in the Hebrew Bible pointing toward this. There are no examples of the mystical-unitive state in the entire text. The problem for the research community, however, is how to incorporate the well-defined cognitive correlates of the prophetic experience—something that is much more difficult to do in the "all is one," "no-self," "no-thought" aspect of the Eastern model. But I believe it can be done, first by characterizing the nature of the interactive-relational state with the same rigor that has been applied to the unitive-mystical one.

Returning to the beings—the cause for this meeting.

The beings may be purely subjective. They may represent our own psychology or, more precisely, the activity of our mind-brain complex. Their nature would be like that of a dream. At the most superficial layer of this model, they may represent residual feelings or thoughts that barely linger in the backs of our minds. At a deeper one, they might be symbolic representations of significant, previously unconscious emotional dynamics. For example, a healing being may represent a health care provider for whom we have strong feelings that we can't express. These psychological notions draw on the implicit assumption of the term *psychedelic*, "mind-manifesting." Our apprehension of the beings reflects or discloses the workings of our mind.

Looking at the beings as objective, we might understand them as residing in alternative levels of reality such as dark matter or parallel universes. Modified consciousness resulting from elevated brain levels of psychedelic compounds, derived from either endogenous or exogenous sources, allows us to peer directly into those realms and view their putative inhabitants.

One approach to determine the objective nature of the beings would be to develop quantum cameras, or dark matter cameras, that allow us to capture images of what exists in these alternative universes. By comparing those images to descriptions of the DMT state, we would be able to determine their correspondence. If they do correspond, we can more confidently posit an external location of the phenomenon.

There's another way to look at the beings as objective, not necessarily as inhabitants of other planets or other planes of existence. They may be sensible representations of normally insensible processes or forces. For example, the beings appear to consist of light, but this may not be their true nature. Instead, "light" might be only the visible representation or manifestation of a particular process. This would be akin to how a flame visibly expresses the operation of combustion. Our perceptual apparatus, as it were, can only see what it is capable of seeing.

What are the external forces that the beings may thus represent? They may include healing and illness, strength and weakness, love and hate, evil and good, wisdom and folly. Using the medieval Jewish philosophers' metaphysics, these are God's intermediaries, the vehicles through which divine efflux or emanation influences the universe, how Providence is effected in the world. For example, apprehension of the activity of the angel Raphael may represent the local action of universal healing forces, and Gabriel those of strength. These world-affecting forces manifest in comprehensible visual, somatic, and other modalities, using the repertoire our minds possess.

This model of the beings adds an additional level of sophistication to a discussion of the objective, externally existent nature of them; that is, they may not be inhabitants of other levels of reality but rather omnipresent forces that exist external to ourselves. These forces we can observe by means of our subjective consciousness. If this is the case, then our invisible world's camera, rather than capturing images of localized objects, may capture images of more pervasive types of forces exerting local effects.

On the other hand, our hypothetical instruments might be unable to capture any images of these external objects or external forces, whether discrete, localized, or local representations of omnipresent forces. This might be the case if perceiving them requires an interaction between them and our minds. In the case of a local manifestation of omnipresent forces, we might theorize that lifeless machines, those without a divinely placed soul, cannot apprehend divine influence. It might simply be too subtle to be objectively recorded. It requires the interaction with a subjectively experienced mind.

This provides a stimulus to expand the field of the term "psychedelic," as I mentioned a few minutes ago. The term may now be invoked to include how our minds apprehend *external* forces that are not being *generated* from within; that is, psychedelic substances may affect how we *perceive* external objects or external forces, as well as how those external objects or forces manifest in our minds. We apprehend the beings in a more or less clear manner depending on the degree of overlay from our own psychology, biology, training, and education. If all of these variables are operating optimally, we apprehend, in as unadulterated a manner as possible, those external things. The less well developed those faculties, the more we muddy our observations with our own internal workings—wishes, hopes, conflicts, and so on. This muddying results in our subjective experience of objective things being more of a mirror and less of a window.

It's never too early to begin thinking about the implications of establishing the reality of the DMT beings. For example, how best to introduce these findings to the public? How will we gauge the value of what the beings share with us? Here we enter into a discussion of true versus false prophecy. To paraphrase Joshua, how can we determine if they are for us or against us? Will we attempt to weaponize them, or will they attempt to weaponize us? Who has access to the beings and for what purposes? There is a host of incalculably complex and ramifying political, religious, ethical, and other issues.

Thanks for listening.*

---

*Because the session ran long, no discussion followed Rick Strassman's presentation due to lack of time.

DAY FOUR

■ ■ ■ ■ ■

Summary and Departure

Over the course of these days, we have attempted to confront assumptions and explore theories about the DMT world. Our discussants, drawn from diverse backgrounds, have challenged each other to consider scientific, environmental, anthropological, psychological, social, spiritual, and artistic perspectives that may enable humanity to shape its future in previously unimagined ways. In our closing remarks, we consider what we know and what we can continue to learn about this mysterious world and its mysterious entities.

CHAPTER 11

What We Think We Know about DMT Entities

DAVID LUKE

First of all, thank you *very* much to Anton for your generosity, your hospitality, and indeed your great vision in bringing this event together. I think something good came of your terrifying encounter experience in that it has enabled this historic event, which has so wonderfully complemented my own vision of bringing the people assembled here together. It has been a great pleasure birthing this symposium with you and with Rory too—it has been great working with you also. It hasn't actually felt like work at all, probably because you did virtually all of the hard work, Rory.

[Audience laughter.]

Thank you too to all the speakers and discussants for coming from all over the world to share your genius with us.

So in our Quest for Truth, what do we know?

Thanks to Dennis [McKenna], concerning DMT, as with other psychedelics, we know some of its chemical characteristics. It is the simplest indole alkaloid, with some curious properties. It has ancient antecedents going back to the origins of multicellular life, if not all life on Earth.

It's not quite a fundamental building block of life; it's a secondary plant compound but one with an extraordinarily broad distribution, occurring widely in mammals, reptiles, fungi —as 4-HO-DMT—and probably all plants, yes, probably *all* plants. Why DMT isn't known to occur in insects is somewhat curious and may say something about why they keep interloping into DMT trips, I don't know.

So while psychedelic plant alkaloids are not primary to life, nature is absolutely drenched in DMT, and at least within plants, such secondary compounds function as endogenous neurotransmitters for "the Gaian mind" by communicating and mediating relationships between species.

As Dennis so elegantly informs us—and as the good prince Peter Kropotkin once did in his famed definition of "anarchy" for the 1910 edition of the *Encyclopaedia Britannica*—Nature operates less by competition and coercion and more by symbiosis, cooperation, mutual aid, and alliances in complex self-organizing communities. These secondary compounds provide the bandwidth for such Gaian telecommunications, although such ideas are only now becoming accepted in the mainstream.

DMT also works as an endogenous neuromodulator within the human nervous system and despite being grossly mislabeled as a neurotoxin is cleanly metabolized and actively transported across the blood-brain barrier and clearly occupies an important position in neural functioning; though what is that function? More on that later.

Meanwhile, back in the lab, DMT's discovery in the developed world extends back a whopping eighty-four years, with [Richard] Manske's first synthesis in 1931, whereas its *indigenous* use in the Americas is far more ancient and extends back at least four thousand years in Tiwanaku. Its *endogenous* use, according to Rick Strassman, could extend back easily as far as the Old Testament and no doubt further. As Andrew Gallimore suggests, it is an ancestral neuromodulator, perhaps once rivaling serotonin as the neurochemical substrate of consciousness, providing the construction materials of our phenomenal and maybe even our noumenal worlds—our very reality. A ground of being, perhaps, with indole foundations providing the extra-dimensional drainage system for Rick's divine overflow. One imagines Soane and Lutyens [the architects of Tyringham Hall] would approve.

Such a combination of the ancestral, the ancient, and the contemporary use of DMT has also embossed a unique and peculiar cultural footprint in the mindscape—as Graham St. John has illustrated—elevating the DMT-pineal near-death hypothesis to iconic status on dance floors and gothic horror cinema screens, the former venerating tryptamine commentators at the peak moment of ecstatic dance frenzies, and the latter extrapolating the meme into grotesque otherworldly jellyfish monstrosities amid zombie serums and cannibalistic pineal-gland-devouring physicians. And yet the actual DMT experience remains even more bizarre and awe inspiring.

Meanwhile [Jeremy] Narby, [Erik] Davis, [Graham] Hancock, and [Ede] Frecska remind us that the DMT experience cannot be wholly understood outside of the cultural context, and yet there are uncanny commonalities at the core of experiences emanating from old folkloric accounts of fairies; anthropological and, indeed, firsthand accounts from indigenous cultures; as well as from FDA-approved experimental research; so-called "recreational" and maybe even biblical DMT trip reports; and even alien abduction cases.

But some sobering warnings apply to the would-be DMT phenomenologist—language is a trap both when deciphering the ineffable and when operating cross-culturally—one man's invisible entity may not be another man's spirit, just as much as a spiritual hierarchy may be orthogonal to horizontal shamanism.

And [Erik] Davis's existential pluralism here should serve to accommodate both the immanent *chthonic animist* beings alongside the transcendent taxonomy of empyrean emissaries. "As above, so sideways," as they say, or as they should say, perhaps.

So that's some of what we know, or we think we know, so what do we believe, or suppose, is actually going on with the DMT experience? We heard from Peter Meyer, who did some of the seminal groundwork in formalizing the question of what might be the nature of these entities.

Like others, he suggests that the DMT experience urges us to go beyond the basic materialistic explanations of reality and explore philosophical and theological positions, as indeed have Rick [Strassman], Erik [Davis], and Rupert [Sheldrake].

Peter's position, like Rick's earlier position, is that DMT could well be the neuromodulating chemical that presides over life and death and that it works as both the midwife and psychopomp of consciousness, leading people into life from a discarnate existence and ushering them back out again when we do the mortal coil shuffle.

This explanation fits well with the data that the DMT space is one that seems highly familiar and that the beings there welcome us back to a carnivalesque world of our youth, populated by cartoonish otherworldly beings and other neonatal atavisms. This is a position that also has accord with the observations of latter-day folklorists— such as anthropologist and former president of the Society for Psychical Research, Andrew Lang—who collected accounts of elven encounters among the Celtic nations of Britain and Ireland.

Lang collected, collated, and published folkloric accounts of the little people spanning a dozen books between 1889 and 1910. He pored over a great many accounts from different cultures from Australia to his native Scotland, and although he refused to believe elves existed, in and of themselves, he instead associated them with phantasms of the dead, particularly with poltergeist phenomena, and thereby associated fairyland with Hades.

Picking up exactly where Lang left off, [Walter] Evans-Wentz was pretty much the next to do the dance around the fairy ring, and he created his magnum opus study on *The Fairy-Faith in Celtic Countries,* published in 1911 [and rereleased in 2004]. Evans-Wentz documented an oral history of the little people across the British Isles and Brittany and discovered that the traditional informants would align the elves with spirits of the dead, although Evans-Wentz himself concluded that they were probably fourth-dimensional beings, existing in what mathematicians had earlier called hyperspace. Although he speculated, like Lang, that this was most likely actually connected to the realm of the dead.

As Evans-Wentz notes [on page 482],

> It is mathematically possible to conceive fourth-dimensional beings, and if they exist it would be impossible in a third-dimensional plane to see them as they really are. Hence the ordinary apparition is non-real as a form, whereas the beings, which wholly sane and reliable seers claim to see when exercising seership of the highest kind, may be as real to themselves and to the seers as human beings are to us here in the third-dimensional world when we exercise normal vision.

This perspective has some resonance with my own observations about the frequently extra-dimensional nature of DMT geometry. [Andrew] Gallimore's perverse metatechnological ontology of the Simulated Universe Theory similarly demands that any artificially intelligent simulated universe, such as our own, must be created by higher-order technologists existing in a world with more dimensions than this one.

Nevertheless, going back to the elves, Evans-Wentz furthermore states that, "Fairyland exists as a supernormal state of consciousness which men and women may enter temporarily in dreams, trances or in various ecstatic conditions, or for an indefinite period at death," which may be a kind of permanent DMT condition.

Such observations, aligning DMT elves with folkloric elves, also resonates with the work of Jacques Vallee and, later, Graham Hancock identifying the parallels among folkloric pixie encounters, DMT dalliances, and alien abduction experiences. Kenneth Ring, the near-death experience [NDE] researcher, also went one step further and indicated how such experience complexes also have great overlap with NDEs.

So one might well be congratulated for supposing, or indeed screaming, the question "Am I dead?" upon first entering the DMT world, as some have been known to do in their first experience.

Rick too, in earlier work, points to the similarity of the NDE to the

DMT experience, although as an alternative Rupert offers up morphic resonance as the means for tuning us in to the NDE.

Graham [Hancock] further observes that the apparent aesthetic manifestation of our systematic ancestral use of altered states—Palaeolithic rock art—also coincided with the technological advances that catalyzed so-called civilization and hints that the more highly advanced alien entities of the DMT world could have been spiking our modulated psyches with sophisticated techne in those moments while drinking deep of altered states. Certainly there are many examples of dreams and psychedelic visions that have given rise to innovation, advanced creativity, and discovery. As Ede Frecska has noted, there has been an important role for visions in shaping all corners of culture.

One good example is the clear biochemical progression from [Dmitri] Mendeleev's dream discovery of the periodic table, through [August] Kekulé's similar dream discovery of the benzene ring structure, [Francis] Crick's possible, though perhaps apocryphal, discovery of the DNA double helix to Kary Mullis's invention of polymerase chain reaction. Alfred Wallace, who Rupert [Sheldrake] speculates may have taken ayahuasca, would no doubt consider such otherworldly intellectual development part of our biologically concomitant spiritual evolution.

So as Graham Hancock rightly notes, with such impediment to important discoveries, might we be stunting our evolution and perhaps "the salvation of the planet *from us*" by prohibiting free access to altered states through drug prohibition?

My own terrifying encounter with someone resembling the angel of death, as indeed many others have seemingly naively done with DMT and similar agents, might deserve attention here [see my article *Disembodied Eyes: An Investigation into Entheogenic Entity Encounters*]. For such divine Promethean characters pop up regularly upon gazing into one's medicine bag for too long or too deeply, and such liminal luminal angelic beings have always been said to have given humans technological secrets. Azreal, the hand of God, whom I may well have met, gave both man the art of blacksmithing and women the art of makeup, according to legend—juxtaposing new crafts for both love and war.

[Peter] Meyer's position on our otherworldly entities is not incongruent with that of Dennis [McKenna], either, who rather than imagining, as does Graham Hancock, that the alien technologies and machinic elves are transdimensional alien beings, speculates that actually *we* are those very alien beings and that the super-advanced futuristic technologies we witness are just that: visions of the future, our *own* future, so that we are the very aliens that abduct us, and we are glimpsing our own genetically engineered extraterrestial selves, who will be needed to fulfill our own Gaian-spermiated otherworldly existence down the line. As [Andrew] Gallimore retorted, we are the DMT aliens, but we have alienated ourselves.

So while DMT entities can be viewed, as Ede [Frecska] does, as quasi-autonomous structures of the nonlocal field—emerging from the nonlocal domains accessible via our intuitive modes of perception—there is facility here for the use of prayer and ritual in guiding these expeditions, as both Rick [Strassman] and Rupert [Sheldrake] advocate in their more theoneurological positions.

As Rupert says, "The potential to participate in the divine mind is always available." And Rick would probably suggest that we merely need to consult our pineal glands and perhaps the Bible too.

For certainly we are in need of road maps here, and if the prophetic experiences of the Old Testament are truly endogenously mediated by DMT, then there may be some tricks we old dogs can learn. One such thing that might be gleaned is how to determine whether such beings are benign or malevolent, especially if Anton's and, indeed, my wife's own experience of being farmed for their emotions by sophisticated overlords is anything to go by.

And yet Erik [Davis] reminds us to always remember that such beings may not always be telling the truth, and he invokes Harner's classic clause regarding the apocalyptic and sinister beings who told him how they had maintained dominion of the universe since the dawn of time, yet the wise old blind shaman shrugged them off nonchalantly for always saying that.

Even so, learning something from [Jeremy] Narby's and indeed [Luis] Luna's anthropological work with the many Amazonian tribes and the oldest known navigators of these worlds, these luminous, shining, blinding, resplendent, and yet ordinarily invisible entities that occupy this other world may well be morally ambiguous, just as humans are. So any such expeditions to see, to know, and to gain power must be mediated by ethics; after all, the Hippocratic oath that governs medicine was born of the dream temple tradition, and indeed Asclepius, the dream healing god who presided over medicine in ancient Greece and Rome and indeed currently here in the West, was as much an endogenous ayahuascero as any shaman or prophet in his semblance as a serpent.

So how to proceed with this pioneering psychonautic endeavor to explore inner space?

We have some canons, traditions, and schools of thought as guides. With such a diverse range of expertise and disciplines as we have here, it serves to observe Erik [Davis's] active agnosticism, lest we throw the molecules, aliens, and divine beings out with the bathwater into the turgid sewers of rigid thinking. Who knows, even some sprinkling of materialism can serve to spice up our beverage with some critical flavor—at least on the biological level—though such spice should be used appropriately; that is, sparingly, and without souring the subtlety of the other fragrant flavors.

So let us proceed with a truly pluralistic and open mind and remember that beliefs are prisons, because our convictions can make us convicts.

Let's start with the pharmacological and experimental means. [Andrew] Gallimore proposes target-controlled continuous IV infusion of DMT sending out intrepid psychonauts for prolonged excursions, perhaps as long as three months—though perhaps he was joking there.

One might think that ayahuasca is a useful substitute, but then there is something in the molecular purity and delivery control prof-fered by Gallimore's bold suggestion here. The ancients have had the inner-space craft built for many millennia already, but what's wrong with applying a few design upgrades from our own culture for good measure?

What are our aims when we get to the point where we can have extended periods of navigation in these realms? Perhaps we can train psychonauts to go on group voyages and somehow remain as a coherent team in the DMT world, as Anton suggests, and then we can begin to explore, communicate with the beings, taxonomize their fauna, set up trade camps, and establish an interdimensional embassy. Echoes are heard here perhaps of [John] Lilly's Earth Coincidence Control Office.

And then what?

Given there are some hard-learned theoretical paradoxes from psychical research about establishing the ontological veracity of dis-carnate beings—given that any new information, technology, or dis-covery supplied by them may actually just be telepathy, clairvoyance, or precognition—might there still be something gained in making such discoveries? We may never be able to ultimately establish where these beings truly exist after all, but something useful may be accomplished along the way.

It's here that the inscription in the Temple of Music truly resonates with what we are doing: "In Quest of Truth—seek truth, but remember that behind all the new knowledge the fundamental issues of life will remain veiled!"

AFTERWORD

What Next?

RORY SPOWERS

Following the success of this first event, the Tyringham Initiative went on to stage another ten events at Tyringham Hall over the following two years, until the house passed into the hands of a new owner in July 2017. Although these events ranged in topics from the entheogenic to the ecological, economic, and educational, all were united by one common quest: to further our understanding of consciousness during this critical time.

A second three-day DMT symposium was held in May 2017, convening eleven new noted speakers in the field along with a new group of discussants drawn from diverse backgrounds. Once again, a series of fascinating presentations emerged from the event, and a number of possible experiments involving DMT were discussed.

Although the Tyringham Initiative is no longer operating from the location where it was born, the project continues to incubate ideas and partner with other organizations within the field to further research and potential methodologies for experimentation. Amid the burgeoning field of new psychedelic research, the exploration of the multidimensional DMT world has only just begun.*

---

*If you would like to be kept informed of progress in this area, please visit www .tyringhaminitiative.com and sign up for free membership.

Speaker Citations

CHAPTER 1

*The Pineal Enigma: The Dazzling Life and
Times of the "Spirit Gland"
—Graham St. John*

Duan, Lia, Omar S. Mabrouk, Tiecheng Liu, et al. "Asphyxia-activated Corticocardiac Signaling Accelerates Onset of Cardiac Arrest." *Proceedings of the National Academy of Sciences of the United States of America* 112, no. 16 (2015): E2073–82.

Leary, Timothy, Ralph Metzner, and Richard Alpert. *The Psychedelic Experience: A Manual Based on the Tibetan Book of the Dead.* New York: University Press Books, 1964.

Lovecraft, Howard Phillips. "From Beyond." *The Fantasy Fan* 1, no. 10 (1934): 147–52.

St. John, Graham. *Mystery School in Hyperspace: A Cultural History of DMT.* New York: Evolver Editions, 2015.

Strassman, Rick. *DMT: The Spirit Molecule: A Doctor's Revolutionary Research into the Biology of Near-death and Mystical Experiences.* Rochester, Vt.: Park Street Press, 2001.

———. "The Pineal Gland: Current Evidence for Its Role in Consciousness." In *Psychedelic Monographs and Essays,* 5th ed., edited by Thomas Lyttle, pages 67–205. Boynton Beach, Fl.: PM & E Publishing Group, 1991.

CHAPTER 2

*Is DMT a Chemical Messenger from an
Extraterrestrial Civilization?*
—Dennis McKenna

Buhner, Stephen Harrod. *Plant Intelligence in the Imaginal Realm: Beyond the Doors of Perception into the Dreaming of the Earth.* Rochester, Vt.: Bear & Company, 2014.

McKenna, Terence. *Food of the Gods: The Search for the Original Tree of Knowledge—A Radical History of Plants, Drugs, and Human Evolution.* New York: Bantam, 1982.

CHAPTER 3

Amazonian Perspectives on Invisible Entities
—Jeremy Narby

Gow, Peter. *Amazonian Myth and Its History.* Oxford: Oxford University Press, 2001.

Kopenawa, Davi, and Bruce Albert. *The Falling Sky: Words of a Yanomami Shaman.* Cambridge, Mass.: Harvard University Press, 2013.

Narby, Jeremy, and Francis Huxley, eds. *Shamans through Time: 500 Years on the Path to Knowledge.* London: Thames and Hudson, 2000.

CHAPTER 4

*Concerning the Nature of the DMT Entities
and Their Relation to Us*
—Peter Meyer

Evans-Wentz, Walter Y. *The Fairy-Faith in Celtic Countries.* Franklin Lakes, N.J.: Career Press, 2004.

Gallimore, Andrew. "Building Alien Worlds: The Neuropsychological and Evolutionary Implications of the Astonishing Psychoactive Effects of *N,N*-dimethyltryptamine (DMT)." *Journal of Scientific Exploration* 27, no. 3 (2013): 455–503.

———. "DMT and the Topology of Reality." In *Neurotransmissions: Psychedelic Essays from Breaking Convention,* edited by Dave King, David Luke, Ben Sessa, Cameron Adams, and Aimee Tollen, pages 9–24. London: Strange Attractor Press, 2015.

Metzinger, Thomas. *The Ego Tunnel: The Science of the Mind and Myth of the Self.* New York: Basic Books, 2009.

Meyer, Peter. "Apparent Communication with Discarnate Entities Induced by Dimethyltryptamine (DMT)." In *Psychedelics,* edited by Thomas Lyttle, pages 161–203. New York: Barricade Books, 1994.

———. "An Essay in the Philosophy of Social Science." Unpublished paper, 1999. http://www.serendipity.li/jsmill/pss2.htm.

———. "340 DMT Trip Reports." 2010. See www.serendipity.li/dmt/340 _dmt_trip_reports.htm. Accessed January 13, 2018.

Moore, Walter J. *A Life of Erwin Schrödinger.* Cambridge: Cambridge University Press, 1994, p. 181.

CHAPTER 5

How to Think about Weird Beings
—Erik Davis

Luhrmann, Tanya M. *When God Talks Back: Understanding the American Evangelical Relationship with God.* New York: Vintage Books, 2012.

CHAPTER 6

Why May DMT Occasion Veridical Hallucinations and
Informative Experiences?
—Ede Frecska

Harner, Michael J. *The Jivaro: People of the Sacred Waterfalls.* Berkeley, Calif.: University of California Press, 1972.

McKenna, Terence. *Food of the Gods: The Search for the Original Tree of Knowledge—A Radical History of Plants, Drugs, and Human Evolution.* New York: Bantam, 1992.

Pitkänen, Matti. *Topological Geometrodynamics.* Bristol, U.K.: Luniver Press, 2006.

Stamets, Paul. *Mycelium Running: How Mushrooms Can Help Save the World.* Berkeley, Calif.: Ten Speed Press, 2005.

Strassman, Rick, Slawek Wojtowicz, Luis Eduardo Luna, and Ede Frecska. *Inner Paths to Outer Space: Journeys to Alien Worlds through Psychedelics and Other Spiritual Technologies.* Rochester, Vt.: Park Street Press, 2008.

CHAPTER 7

The Neurobiology of Conscious Interaction with
Alternate Realities and Their Inhabitants
—Andrew Gallimore

Gallimore, Andrew. "Building Alien Worlds: The Neuropsychological and Evolutionary Implications of the Astonishing Psychoactive Effects of *N,N*-dimethyltryptamine (DMT)." *Journal of Scientific Exploration* 27, no. 3 (2013): 455–503.

Gallimore, Andrew, and Rick Strassman. "A Model for the Application of Target-controlled Intravenous Infusion for a Prolonged Immersive Psychedelic Experience." *Frontiers in Pharmacology* 7, no. 211 (2016): 1–11.

Hesse, Hermann. *Demian.* Berlin: Fischer Verlag, 1919.

Kastrup, Bernardo. *Why Materialism Is Baloney: How True Skeptics Know There Is No Death and Fathom Answers to Life, the Universe, and Everything.* Southampton, U.K.: Iff Books, 2014.

CHAPTER 8

Morphic Resonance, Psychedelic Experience,
and Collective Memory
—Rupert Sheldrake

Carr, Bernard. *Universe or Multiverse?* Cambridge: Cambridge University Press, 2010.

Fox, Matthew, and Rupert Sheldrake. *The Physics of Angels: Exploring the Realm Where Science and Spirit Meet.* Rhinebeck, N.Y.: Monkfish Book Publishing Company, 2014.

Hart, David Bentley. *The Experience of God: Being, Consciousness, Bliss.* New Haven, Conn.: Yale University Press, 2014.

Sheldrake, Rupert. *A New Science of Life,* 3rd ed. London: Icon Books, 2009.

Wallace, Alfred Russel. *The World of Life: A Manifestation of Creative Power, Directive Mind and Ultimate Purpose.* London: Chapman & Hall, 1914.

CHAPTER 9

Psychedelics, Entities, Dark Matter, and Parallel Dimensions
—Graham Hancock

Crick, Francis. *Life Itself: Its Origin and Nature.* London: Futura, 1982.

Hancock, Graham, ed. *Divine Spark: Psychedelics, Consciousness and the Birth of Civilization.* London: Hay House, 2005.

————. *Supernatural: Meetings with the Ancient Teachers of Mankind.* London: Century, 2005.

Vallee, Jacques. *Passport to Magonia.* Chicago: Henry Regnery Company, 1969.

CHAPTER 11

What We Think We Know about DMT Entities
—David Luke

Evans-Wentz, Walter Y. *The Fairy-faith in Celtic Countries.* Franklin Lakes, N.J.: Career Press, 2004.

Gallimore, Andrew, and David Luke. "DMT Research from 1956 to the End of Time." In *Neurotransmissions: Psychedelic Essays from Breaking Convention,* edited by Dave King, Ben Sessa, Cameron Adams, and Aimee Tollen, pages 291–316. London: Strange Attractor Press, 2015.

Luke, David. "Discarnate Entities and Dimethyltryptamine (DMT): Psycho-pharmacology, Phenomenology and Ontology." *Journal of the Society for Psychical Research* 75 (2011): 26–42.

————. "Disembodied Eyes Revisited: An Investigation into the Ontology of Entheogenic Entity Encounters." *Entheogen Review: The Journal of Unauthorized Research on Visionary Plants and Drugs* 17, no. 1 (2008): 1–9 & 38–40 (article references).

————. "Rock Art or Rorschach: Is There More to Entoptics Than Meets the Eye?" *Time & Mind: The Journal of Archaeology, Consciousness & Culture* 3 (2010): 9–28.

————. "So Long as You've Got Your Elf: Death, DMT and Discarnate Entities." In *Daimonic Imagination: Uncanny Intelligence,* edited by Angela Voss and William Rowlandson, pages 282–91. Cambridge: Cambridge Scholars Publishing, 2013.

Speaker Biographies

Erik Davis, Ph.D., is an author, podcaster, and award-winning journalist and media critic based in San Francisco. His wide-ranging work focuses on the intersection of alternative religion, media, and the popular imagination. He is the author, most recently, of *Nomad Codes: Adventures in Modern Esoterica*. He also wrote *The Visionary State: A Journey through California's Spiritual Landscape*, and *TechGnosis: Myth, Magic, and Mysticism in the Age of Information*, which has been translated into five languages. He also wrote a short critical volume on Led Zeppelin. His essays on music, technoculture, and spirituality have appeared in dozens of books, including *Sound Unbound, AfterBurn: Reflections on Burning Man, Zig Zag Zen,* and *Rave Culture and Religion*. Davis has contributed to scores of publications, including *Bookforum, Salon, Slate, Artforum, Wired,* the *LA Weekly,* and the *Village Voice.* He appears in numerous documentaries and has been interviewed by CNN, the BBC, public radio, and the *New York Times.* For over five years, he has been exploring the "cultures of consciousness" on his weekly podcast *Expanding Mind* on the Progressive Radio Network. He graduated from Yale University in 1988 and recently earned his Ph.D. in religious studies from Rice University.

Ede Frecska, Ph.D., is chairman of the department of psychiatry at the University of Debrecen, Hungary. He received his medical degree in 1977 from the Semmelweis University in Hungary. He then earned qualifications as a certified psychologist from the department of psychology at Eötvös Loránd University in Budapest. Frecska completed his residency training in psychiatry both in Hungary and in the United States. He is a qualified psychopharmacologist of international merit with seventeen years of clinical and research experience in the United States. During his early academic years, Frecska's studies were devoted to research on schizophrenia and affective illness. He published more than fifty scientific papers and book chapters on these topics. In his recent research he is engaged in studies on psychointegrator plants and techniques. He is particularly interested in the physiological role of endohallucinogen compounds (DMT, 5MeO-DMT, and bufotenin). Frecska is a member of several professional organizations and has received grants and awards from a variety of sources.

Andrew Gallimore, Ph.D., is a neurobiologist, pharmacologist, and chemist currently based at the Okinawa Institute of Science and Technology, where he develops computational models of the signaling pathways underlying neural functions. He has been interested in the neural basis of psychedelic drug action for many years and is the author of a number of articles on DMT and the psychedelic state, including "Building Alien Worlds," in which he developed a new model of DMT's effects on neural function and its relationship to human neuroevolution. He recently published the first theoretical paper to link the phenomenology of the psychedelic state to Giulio Tononi's integrated information theory (IIT) of consciousness. He is also currently collaborating with David Luke to perform the first detailed phenomenological analysis of the subjective reports (bedside notes) of the sixty volunteers in Rick Strassman's landmark human DMT study. It is hoped that this work will further our understanding of the ontological significance of the astonishing psychoactive effects of this unique psychedelic.

Graham Hancock is the author of the major international nonfiction bestsellers *The Sign and the Seal, Fingerprints of the Gods, The Message of the Sphinx, Heaven's Mirror, Underworld,* and *Supernatural* and of the epic adventure novels *Entangled* and *War God.* His books have sold more than seven million copies worldwide and have been translated into thirty languages. His public lectures, radio, and TV appearances, including two major TV series—*Quest for the Lost Civilization* and *Underworld: Flooded Kingdoms of the Ice Age*—as well as his strong presence on the internet have put his ideas before tens of millions. He has become recognized as an unconventional thinker who raises resonant questions about humanity's past and about our present predicament. In February 2015 Hancock was voted No. 30 in the Watkins' list of "The 100 Most Spiritually Influential Living People." Hancock's newest book is titled *Magicians of the Gods.*

Dennis McKenna, Ph.D., has pursued interdisciplinary research in the study of Amazonian ethnopharmacology and plant hallucinogens for over thirty years. He has conducted extensive ethnobotanical fieldwork in the Peruvian, Colombian, and Brazilian Amazon, recently completing a four-year project investigating Amazonian ethnomedicines as potential treatments for cognitive deficits. His doctoral research (University of British Columbia, 1984) focused on the ethnopharmacology of ayahuasca and *oo-koo-he,* two tryptamine-based hallucinogens used by indigenous peoples in the northwest Amazon. McKenna completed postdoctoral research fellowships in neurosciences in the Laboratory of Clinical Pharmacology at the National Institute of Mental Health (1986–88), and in the department of neurology at the Stanford University School of Medicine (1988–90). He joined Shaman Pharmaceuticals as director of ethnopharmacology in 1990, and subsequently joined Aveda Corporation as senior research pharmacognosist. He is currently an assistant professor in the Center for Spirituality and Healing at the University of Minnesota, where he teaches courses in ethnopharmacology, botanical medicines, and plants in human affairs.

He is a founding board member of the Heffter Research Institute, a nonprofit research organization focused on the development of therapeutic applications for psychedelic medicines. He was a key organizer and participant in the Hoasca Project, the first biomedical investigation of ayahuasca used sacramentally by the UDV, a Brazilian religious sect. McKenna is author or coauthor of four books and over fifty scientific papers in peer-reviewed journals.

Peter Meyer majored in philosophy and mathematics and worked from 1980 to 1994 in California as a computer programmer and software developer. There he met Terence McKenna and collaborated with him in developing the software to illustrate his Timewave Zero theory. Pursuing his early established interest in psychedelic exploration, in 1993 he published the first article describing in detail contact with intelligent entities in the DMT space. He conducted postgraduate research in computational physics at the University of Derby and in 2000 received an MPhil degree for this work. Since 2001 he has made his living as an independent software developer and publisher while traveling in Europe, Asia, Africa, and South America. In 2010 he began to develop computational astrology software inspired by the work of Richard Tarnas. His interests include philosophy, history, classical music, and opera, and especially the current global geopolitical situation and its background.

Jeremy Narby, Ph.D., is an anthropologist and writer who grew up in Canada and Switzerland. He studied history at the University of Canterbury, receiving a doctorate in anthropology from Stanford University. Narby spent several years living with the Asháninka tribe in the Peruvian Amazon, cataloging indigenous uses of rainforest resources. Experiences with ayahuasca during his research inspired his first book, *The Cosmic Serpent: DNA and the Origins of Knowledge*. In the book, Narby proposes that indigenous people have developed a deep understanding of medicinal plants and even DNA itself through ritualized use of ayahuasca, a theory deemed heretical by mainstream science. Jeremy has since written three other books: *Shamans through Time: 500 Years on the Path to Knowledge, Intelligence in Nature,* and *The Psychotropic Mind: The World According to Ayahuasca, Iboga, and Shamanism.* He lectures worldwide and sponsors rain forest expeditions for biologists and other scientists to examine indigenous knowledge systems and the utility of ayahuasca in gaining knowledge. He was featured in the documentary *DMT: The Spirit Molecule.* Since 1989, Narby has been working as the Amazonian projects director for the Swiss NGO, Nouvelle Planète.

Rupert Sheldrake, Ph.D., is a biologist and author of more than eighty scientific papers and ten books. He was among the top one hundred Global Thought Leaders for 2013, as ranked by the Duttweiler Institute, Switzerland's leading think tank. A scholar of Clare College, he studied natural sciences at Cambridge University. He then studied philosophy and history of science at Harvard before returning to Cambridge, where he completed a Ph.D. in biochemistry and became director of studies in biochemistry and cell biology. While at Cambridge, together with Philip Rubery, he discovered the mechanism of polar auxin transport. He has studied rain forest plants in Kuala Lumpur, Malaysia, and was principal plant physiologist and consultant physiologist at the International Crops Research Institute for the Semi-Arid Tropics in Hyderabad, India, where he helped develop new cropping systems now widely used. While in India, he also lived at the ashram of Father Bede Griffiths, where he wrote his first book, *A New Science of Life.*

Since 1981, he has continued research on developmental and cell biology. He has also investigated unexplained aspects of animal behavior and similar phenomena in people, which is summarized in his books *Seven Experiments That Could Change the World, Dogs That Know When Their Owners Are Coming Home,* and *The Sense of Being Stared At.*

In his 2012 book called *The Science Delusion* in the United

Kingdom and *Science Set Free* in the United States, he examines ten dogmas of modern science and shows how, as questions, they open up new vistas of scientific possibility.

Graham St. John, Ph.D., is an Australian cultural anthropologist specializing in entheogens, dance music cultures, and neotribes. He has written several books, including *Mystery School in Hyperspace: A Cultural History of DMT, Global Tribe: Technology, Spirituality and Psytrance,* and *Technomad: Global Raving Countercultures.* He has held fellowships in Australia, the United States, Canada, and Switzerland. He recently began researching the global Burning Man diaspora in Europe. A frequent speaker at conferences and transformational festivals, he is the founding executive editor of *Dancecult: Journal of Electronic Dance Music Culture.*

Rick Strassman, M.D., obtained his undergraduate degree in biological sciences from Stanford University and his medical degree from the Albert Einstein College of Medicine of Yeshiva University. He trained in general psychiatry at the University of California, Davis, in Sacramento and took a clinical psychopharmacology research fellowship at the University of California, San Diego. Joining the faculty at the University of New Mexico in 1984, he first studied pineal melatonin function in humans. From 1990 to 1995 he performed the first new clinical research with psychedelic drugs in the United States in a generation, focusing primarily on DMT and psilocybin, receiving funding from the National Institute on Drug Abuse and the Scottish Rite Schizophrenia Research Foundation. In 2007, he cofounded the Cottonwood Research Foundation with Andrew Stone and Steven Barker. He has authored or coauthored over thirty-five peer-reviewed scientific papers and served as a consultant to various government, nonprofit, and for-profit entities. His book *DMT: The Spirit Molecule* has sold 150,000 copies, has been translated into twelve languages, and is the basis of a successful independent documentary that he coproduced. He is coauthor of *Inner Paths to Outer Space* and is the author of *DMT and the Soul of Prophecy*. He is currently a clinical associate professor of psychiatry at the University of New Mexico School of Medicine.

Discussant Biographies

Robin Carhart-Harris, Ph.D., successfully coordinated the first clinical study of psilocybin in the United Kingdom and the first clinical study of a classic psychedelic drug in the UK for over forty years. After being awarded a master's of art in psychoanalysis at Brunel University, London, Carhart-Harris completed his Ph.D. in psychopharmacology at the University of Bristol. In 2009, under the mentorship of professor David Nutt, Carhart-Harris moved to Imperial College London to continue his fMRI research with the classic psychedelic drug psilocybin. Over the last four years Carhart-Harris and Nutt have built a program of research with psychedelics that includes fMR and magnetoencephalography (MEG) imaging with psilocybin, fMR imaging with MDMA, and soon a clinical trial sponsored by the Medical Research Council to assess the efficacy of psilocybin as a treatment for major depression. Carhart-Harris has articles published in *Brain,* the *Proceedings of the National Academy of Sciences,* and the *British Journal of Psychiatry* with several other relevant papers to follow. Carhart-Harris has been supported by the Beckley Foundation, the Neuropsychoanalysis Foundation, the Heffter Research Institute, and the Multidisciplinary Association for Psychedelic Studies.

Bernard Carr, Ph.D., studied mathematics as an undergraduate at Trinity College, Cambridge. For his Ph.D. he studied the first second of the Universe, working under Stephen Hawking. He was elected to a fellowship at Trinity in 1975, and in 1980 he became a senior research fellow at the Institute of Astronomy in Cambridge. In 1985 he moved to Queen Mary College, University of London, where he is now professor of mathematics and astronomy. He has also held visiting professorships at various institutes in America, Canada, and Japan. His professional area of research is cosmology and relativity, with particular interest in such topics as the early universe, black holes, dark matter, and the anthropic principle. He has recently edited the book *Universe or Multiverse?* He also has a longstanding interest in the interface between science and religion, having recently contributed an article on cosmology and religion to *The Oxford Handbook of Religion and Science.*

Vimal Darpan weaves thirty years of experience in music, healing, and the shamanic arts to create a unique transmission that inspires, enlivens, and transforms. His home is in Australia, where he is renowned as a teacher, musician, and healer. Bringing people together to create an unambiguous experience of our common Source is the intention that inspires his work, which uses a skillful blend of ceremony, song, meditation, and celebration. Darpan is a spontaneous and engaging speaker with a natural flair for embellishing his talks with interesting stories, anecdotal references, and rich personal experience. He delivers a wealth of information within a context that inspires and motivates. His passion is creating positive change by initiating vision and awakening new perspectives. Darpan is currently working on a book that references his many years of experience in the shamanic and healing arts, and he is available to deliver talks, concerts, seminars, and workshops anywhere in the world.

Santha Faiia is a professional photographer specializing in ancient cultures and monuments. Her work has been published around the world in major newspapers and magazines, and in 1990, her photographic exhibition *Ethiopian Trilogy* was opened at the Royal Geographical Society London by Her Royal Highness Princess Anne. Faiia's work illustrated *The Sign and the Seal* and *Fingerprints of the Gods,* and in 1998 her major book of photographs was published—the international bestseller *Heaven's Mirror.* Faiia's images from sacred sites as far afield as the temples of Angkor in Cambodia and the great pyramids of Giza in Egypt bring to life a lost world and "achieve the rare feat of making you feel you are there" (*Western Mail*). Faiia worked closely with Graham Hancock on *Underworld.* Her photographs of the many ancient underwater ruins—off the coast of Japan, all around the Pacific, off Indonesia and Malaysia, off India, and in the Mediterranean, the Atlantic, and the Caribbean—add a whole new dimension to her work. She also photographed *Supernatural,* putting unique images of the ancient rock art of South Africa before a global public. In 2013, Faiia's photographs of Easter Island were presented at the Vatican Ethnological Museum, supporting a special exhibition of Easter Island artifacts. In 2014 a second exhibition at the Vatican Ethnological Museum, this time on Indonesia, was again accompanied by a collection of Faiia's photographs. Faiia's latest work is to be seen in the thirty-two pages of color photographs she has contributed to the forthcoming *Magicians of the Gods.*

Amanda Feilding, Countess of Wemyss and March, is a British scientist and founding director of the Beckley Foundation, a UN accredited NGO aimed toward reforming drug policy. The Beckley Foundation is dedicated to providing a rigorous, independent review of global drug policy in an effort to reduce the harms associated with both the misuse of drugs and the policies that aim to control them. The intention of the foundation is to help develop policies that are evidence based and rational. To this end, Feilding has hosted many influential seminars on international drug policy. Bringing together leading academics, experts, and policy makers from around the world, these seminars initiate such innovations as the call for a drug classification system based on a scientifically evaluated scale of harm. Fascinated by mysticism and states of altered consciousness since childhood, Feilding famously gained notoriety in 1970 when she documented her own trepanation in the film *Heartbeat in the Brain,* then subsequently in a 1998 documentary, *A Hole in the Head.* In *Blood and Consciousness,* Feilding also published her own theories about how trepanation influences blood-oxygen levels in the brain and can create an expansion in consciousness.

Anna Hope is a novelist and nonfiction writer. She was educated at Oxford University, RADA, The University of London, and in various jungles and deserts in central and south America. Her fiction has been translated into ten languages and has been short-listed for numerous prizes. She was visiting fellow at the University of Essex, where she lectured on Rebecca Solnit and the Politics of Uncertainty.

Luis Eduardo Luna, Ph.D., is an anthropologist and noted ayahuasca researcher. Luna was born in 1947 in Florencia, Colombia. He received his doctorate in 1989 from the Institute of Comparative Religion at Stockholm University as well as an honorary doctorate in 2000 from St. Lawrence University, New York. He is currently a language teacher at the Swedish School of Economics and Business Administration in Helsinki, Finland. Luna is best known for his research on the entheogenic tea ayahuasca. His research has focused on traditional indigenous usage as well as the newer syncretic ayahuasca churches such as Santo Daime and the União do Vegetal. He is the director of Wasiwaska—Research Centre for the Study of Psychointegrator Plants, Visionary Art, and Consciousness, located in Brazil; currently, they are studying the neurological aspects of ayahuasca inebriation on the central nervous system.

Cosmo Feilding Mellen started directing documentaries after graduating from Oxford University in 2008. His first feature documentary was *Breaking the Taboo,* narrated by Morgan Freeman and featuring interviews with Bill Clinton, Jimmy Carter, and other presidents from around the world. The film was an exposé of the failed international War on Drugs. His second documentary feature, *The Sunshine Makers,* was produced by Academy Award–winning Passion Pictures and tells the story of two underground chemists who tried to save the world with LSD and in the process fueled the psychedelic revolution of the 1960s.

Jill Purce is a British voice teacher, Family Constellations therapist, and author. In the 1970s Purce developed a new way of working with the voice, introducing the teaching of group overtone chanting, producing a single note while amplifying vocal harmonics. Between 1971 and 1974 she lived and worked in Germany with the composer Karlheinz Stockhausen. Since the early 1970s she has taught internationally diverse forms of contemplative chant, particularly overtone chanting. For over fifteen years she has been leading Family Constellations combined with chant. She is the author of *The Mystic Spiral: Journey of the Soul,* a book about the spiral in sacred traditions, art, and psychology; as well as numerous articles. She is a former fellow of King's College London, biophysics department, and has produced over thirty books as general editor of the Thames and Hudson Art and Imagination series.

Will Rowlandson is senior lecturer in hispanic studies at the University of Kent. He has published on various areas of Latin American studies, including the history of Guantánamo Bay detention center's use of rendition and torture during the War on Terror. He also teaches aspects of Latin American cultural history, including the prose and poetry of Borges, Lezama Lima, Cabrera Infante, and Rulfo, as well as Cuban literature and film of the revolutionary era.

Tony Wright is a consciousness researcher based in Penzance, Cornwall, who studied horticulture and plant biochemistry at the Royal Botanic

Garden in Edinburgh. He is the coauthor with Graham Gynn of *Return to the Brain of Eden: Restoring the Connection between Neurochemistry and Consciousness,* an acclaimed study of the transgenerational epigenetic theory of evolution and its impact on the development of the human brain.

Editor and Symposium
Curator Biographies

Anton Bilton (Host) is an economics graduate from City, University of London. He was the founder of The Raven Group and has also been a founder and director of three other companies that have floated on the London stock exchange's Alternative Investment Market (AIM). He is currently executive deputy chairman of Raven Russia Limited. Outside of his working environment, Anton's principal interest is altered states of consciousness and entheogenic plant sentience.

David Luke, Ph.D., (Moderator/Curator) is a senior lecturer in psychology at the University of Greenwich, where he teaches an undergraduate course on the psychology of exceptional human experience. His research focuses on transpersonal experiences, anomalous phenomena, and altered states of consciousness, especially via psychedelics, having published more than one hundred academic papers in this area, including eight books, most recently *Neurotransmissions: Essays on Psychedelics* and *Talking with the Spirits: Ethnographies from between the Worlds.* Luke is also director of the Ecology, Cosmos and Consciousness salon at the Institute of Ecotechnics, London, and is a cofounder and director of Breaking Convention: International Conference on Psychedelic Consciousness. He has studied techniques of consciousness alteration from South America to India from the perspective of scientists, shamans, and Shivaites and lives life on the edge of Sussex, UK.

Rory Spowers (Curator/Coordinator) is an ecological writer, campaigner, and filmmaker who moved from mid-Wales to Sri Lanka in 2004 and has been living in Ibiza since 2012, where he first went to work with BBC presenter Bruce Parry on the feature film *Quest*. Rory's last book, *A Year in Green Tea and Tuk Tuks*, covers the creation of Samakanda "Bio-versity," an ecological learning center in south Sri Lanka. His previous book *Rising Tides* was a history of ecological thought and was critically acclaimed by the UK *Sunday Times*, the *Observer*, and a variety of magazines. Rory's first book, *Three Men on a Bike*, follows a bizarre cycling trip through Africa with friends on the original three-seater *trandem* used by *The Goodies* on BBC TV in the 1970s. In 2002 Rory founded The Web of Hope, a UK charity and ecological education resource highlighting role models for sustainability, social justice, and positive change, now part of Sustainapedia. Most recently, he has been working with Mangu TV promoting documentary films such as *Neurons to Nirvana—Understanding Psychedelic Medicines*. He is a curator for The Tyringham Project.

Index

Crick, Francis, 157, 255, 256–57
cross-cultural influences. *See also* shaman
    cultural overlay on entities, 86–87, 299
    DMT experience in context of, 299
    pop culture about DMT, 16–25, 299
    rituals and cultural memory, 211–12

darkness, 34–35, 36, 186, 259–60
Darpan, Vimal, 30, 84–85, 92, 198,
    263, 321
Darwin's Pharmacy (Doyle), 144
Davis, Erik, 27–28, 68, 93–94,
    118–53, 203–4, 238–39, 268,
    299, 300, 303, 304, 313
Dawkins, Richard, 228, 274
death
    awareness of DMT World near, 112
    examining dying brain for DMT,
    29–31
    Sheldrake's theories of after, 215–17
de Chardin, Pierre Teilhard, 189
DeKorne, Jim, 171–72
Demian (Hesse), 176
Descartes, René, 13, 32, 99, 167, 189
Diaz, Carlos, 247
dimethyltryptamine. *See* DMT
Disembodied Eyes (Luke), 302
Divine Spark, The (Hancock), 245
"DMT and the Topology of Reality"
    (Gallimore), 104, 108–9
DMT (dimethyltryptamine). *See also*
    endogenous DMT; entities
    as ancestral neuromodulator, 103,
    113, 184, 298
    chemical properties of, 38–42, 297–98
    common occurrence of, 46–48
    effects on body, 276
    exploring reality using, 7
    found in dying brain, 29–31
    history of studies about, 275–76
    implied reductionism in study of, 82
    increasing sonically, 31–32

intermediary function of, 142
IV infusion of, 195–96, 198–200,
    266, 304–5
measuring endogenous, 33–34
multidisciplinary research of,
    118–19
neuromodulation properties of,
    102–3, 298
as neurotransmitter, 12
origins and phylogeny of, 53–54, 55
pop culture about, 19–25, 299
role in neural evolution, 56–57
shamanistic use of, 49–50
sleep deprivation and, 34
spiritual quality of, 141–42
symposia on, 307
trees bearing, 26, 27
urban myths of, 275
user experiences of, 9, 10, 51–52,
    214, 242–45, 253–54, 302
vestigial uses of, 185
DMT: The Spirit Molecule
    (Strassman), 8, 10–11, 247
DMT World
    awareness at death of, 112
    chemical changes and perception of,
    279–80
    childhood motifs in, 114
    defined, 95–96, 102
    disincarnate entities in, 100–101,
    300
    flora and fauna of, 267
    Hebraic model of, 279–80, 281–84
    links to fetal brain, 105–6, 110
    phenomenal vs. noumenal worlds,
    108–9
    reality of, 197, 277–81
    research descriptions of, 276–77
    survival value of building, 104–5
    Zen models of, 278–79, 280, 281
DNA molecule, 255, 257–58
Doyle, Richard, 144